DIABETES IN ELDERLY PEOPLE

DIABETES IN ELDERLY PEOPLE

A guide for the health care team

Edited by
COLIN M. KESSON,
Consultant Physician and Diabetologist,
Victoria Infirmary,
Glasgow

and

PAUL V. KNIGHT,
Consultant Physician in Geriatric Medicine,
Lightburn General Hospital,
Glasgow

Chapman and Hall
London · New York · Tokyo · Melbourne · Madras

UK	Chapman and Hall, 11 New Fetter Lane, London EC4P 4EE
USA	Chapman and Hall, 29 West 35th Street, New York NY10001
JAPAN	Chapman and Hall Japan, Thomson Publishing Japan, Hirakawacho Nemoto Building, 7F, 1–7–11 Hirakawa-cho, Chiyoda-ku, Tokyo 102
AUSTRALIA	Chapman and Hall Australia, Thomas Nelson Australia, 480 La Trobe Street, PO Box 4725, Melbourne 3000
INDIA	Chapman and Hall India, R. Sheshadri, 32 Second Main Road, CIT East, Madras 600 035

First edition

© 1990 Chapman and Hall

Typeset in 11/12 Sabon by Scarborough Typesetting Services
Printed in Great Britain by St Edmundsbury Press,
Bury St Edmunds, Suffolk

ISBN 0 412 32870 4

British Library Cataloguing in Publication Data

Diabetes in elderly people.
 1. Old persons. Diabetes
 I. Kesson, C. M. II. Knight P. V.
 618.97'6462

 ISBN 0–412–32870–4

Library of Congress Cataloging-in-Publication Data available

CONTENTS

CONTRIBUTORS

Francis I. Caird MA DM FRCP
(Lond. and Glasg.)
David Cargill Professor of Geriatric Medicine, University of Glasgow, Glasgow, UK

Colin M. Kesson MBChB MRCP
Consultant Physician and Diabetologist, Victoria Infirmary, Glasgow, UK

Paul V. Knight MBChB MRCP
Consultant Physician in Geriatric Medicine, Lightburn Hospital, Glasgow; Visiting Assistant Professor of Medicine, North Eastern Ohio Universities College of Medicine, USA

Brendan J. Martin MBChB MRCP
Consultant Physician in Geriatric Medicine, Lightburn Hospital, Glasgow, UK

Kenneth R. Paterson MBChB MRCP
Consultant Physician and Diabetologist, Royal Infirmary and Southern General Hospital, Glasgow, UK

Patricia A. Phillips SRD
Dietitian, Victoria Infirmary, Glasgow, UK

Maureen Roberts RGN SCM
Diabetic Liaison Sister, Victoria Infirmary, Glasgow, UK

ACKNOWLEDGEMENTS

We are greatly indebted to our secretaries, Miss Lorraine Mitchell and Mrs Mary Gibb, as well as to all the contributors for their patience and effort. We would also like to thank our publishers for their good advice, and Mr John Main of the medical illustration department of the Victoria Infirmary for his excellent illustrations.

Colin M. Kesson
Paul V. Knight

PREFACE

This book is intended for all members of the health care team who look after elderly people with diabetes mellitus. This includes specialist nurses in diabetes and care of the elderly, other nurses who might be involved with elderly diabetic patients, hospital doctors, general practitioners, dietitians, and other paramedical staff as well as students in these various disciplines.

It is not an exhaustive text, but includes plenty of background references for those who wish to pursue a topic further.

FOREWORD

It has been said that old age is not so bad when you consider the alternative; but, fortunately on occasion symptoms attributed to ageing are due to treatable disease. This useful book draws attention to diabetes mellitus, a common illness in elderly people, which can cause serious disability and should be diagnosed promptly and treated correctly. In this text the facts are well documented that the diagnosis may alarm old people and thus a full explanation must be given and the likely benefits of an adequate therapeutic regimen described.

Drs Paul Knight and Colin Kesson are physicians intimately concerned with the day to day diagnosis and treatment of diabetes and they have enlisted the assistance of colleagues of outstanding ability, thus demonstrating the vital importance of teamwork in the control of this disease.

Modern geriatric practice is proving of inestimable value to older people and detailed accounts such as this, of the practical comprehensive management of an illness, show that while diagnosis is still fundamental, the essential components of complete empathy with the patient as a whole person and continuity of care are essential to obtain good results. Education of elderly people with diabetes, dietary assessment and therapy, appropriate medication and important complications are subjects clearly discussed, with detailed guidance given.

We live in a world in which the lifespan of the population is increasing steadily and the numbers of elderly people growing, thus knowledge must increase to help every old person to enjoy these added years. I am therefore delighted to be invited to introduce this most helpful addition to the constantly improving literature of geriatric medicine, which without doubt will enhance the quality of life of many older citizens.

Sir W. Ferguson Anderson
Emeritus Professor of Geriatric Medicine
Glasgow University

INTRODUCTION
A short guide to some salient points

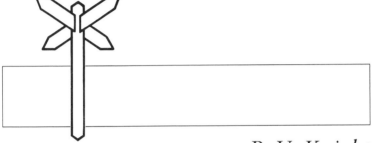

P. V. Knight
and
C. M. Kesson

NUMBERS AND PRESENTATION

Remember that diabetes is common in the elderly population, afflicting as many as 1 in 10.

Diabetes may produce a substantial amount of disability and is therefore worth treating seriously.

Many elderly patients may have no symptoms initially, or present with one of the 'geriatric giants' viz., immobility (because of peripheral vascular disease), instability (because of postural hypotension), urinary incontinence (because of osmotic diuresis) and intellectual deterioration (because of incipient coma).

Other elderly patients may present with complications of diabetes which are incorrectly ascribed to old age, e.g. failing eyesight secondary to retinopathy.

Random blood glucose and glycosylated haemoglobin tests are worthwhile screening procedures in any ill elderly patient.

EDUCATION AND DIET

Education and diet are the cornerstones of therapy.

Dietary therapy should not be forgotten, by staff or patients, when some other treatment, e.g. an oral hypoglycaemic, is commenced. It must be individually tailored; diet sheets handed out without explanation will almost certainly not be adhered to.

Most elderly patients have very poor comprehension of the various facets of diabetes, but most are willing to try to learn when given the opportunity.

Education of the elderly patient may be best carried out by a specialist nurse with whom the patient may more easily identify. It should be planned and not take place haphazardly.

PHARMACOLOGICAL THERAPY

Oral therapy should only be commenced when it is certain that an adequate trial of dietary therapy has failed. A short acting oral agent is to be preferred.

Insulin therapy should be commenced for the same good clinical reasons as in younger patients. A once daily injection of insulin may be adequate for symptomatic control. Less than 3% of elderly patients receiving insulin will need the services of the community nurse to administer the injection. Injection aids may be considered, to enhance independence.

MONITORING THERAPY

Self monitoring of any hypoglycaemic therapy is best done by means of capillary glucose testing, particularly in those patients on insulin or drugs. Instructions for any monitoring procedure should be carefully explained and demonstrated and their significance emphasized.

FOOT CARE

Foot problems are common and often lead to serious disability, particularly in an elderly population who may have co-existing difficulties in looking after their own feet. Regular foot inspection is vital. Penetrating foot lesions should always be referred early for specialist opinion.

PRESCRIBING DIFFICULTIES

Prescribing for the elderly person with diabetes should take into account the ability of the patient to comply with therapy. The prescriber should remember the hazards of polypharmacy, the effect the drugs will have on the blood glucose and the patient's response to hypoglycaemia.

Prescribing more than three medicines for any elderly person may result in none of the drugs being taken correctly.

Proprietary medicines which contain sugar are not too troublesome, provided they are not taken over a prolonged period or to excess.

HYPOGLYCAEMIA AND HYPERGLYCAEMIA

Symptoms of hypoglycaemia may be very vague and chronic hypoglycaemia might be mistaken for a dementing process. Acute hypoglycaemia can result in fatality and is usually a result of a mismatch of therapy and dietary intake.

It is almost never correct to stop hypoglycaemic therapy during illness. Often there is an increased requirement.

Patients should not be encouraged to allow chronic hyperglycaemia as they often feel non-specifically unwell because of this, and it encourages the development of complications. Hyperglycaemia may complicate any intercurrent illness.

COMPLICATIONS OF DIABETES

Monitoring for complications must be undertaken on a regular and systematic basis by trained personnel. Early detection of complications may prevent much disability and morbidity.

SHARING CARE BETWEEN HOSPITAL AND COMMUNITY

Shared care of diabetic patients requires the enthusiastic participation of all the team members.

Ideally, many elderly people with diabetes can be cared for by their own family doctors, but successful management often requires more time than allotted to the normal consultation.

A practice of less than 5000 patients will probably not have enough diabetic patients to make a mini-clinic worthwhile.

1

EPIDEMIOLOGY AND PATHOPHYSIOLOGY
Who, where, what and why?

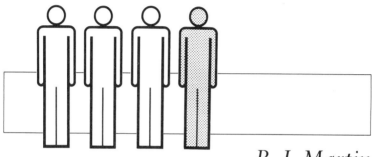

B. J. Martin
and
P. V. Knight

WHO AND WHERE?

Diabetes mellitus is a worldwide health problem, but prevalence rates vary greatly between different societies and ethnic groups. In the industrialized nations, such as the USA and those of western Europe, the prevalence is approximately 2% among young adults and 15% in those aged over 65 years; but in developing countries the disease is less common, with overall rates averaging 1%. It is likely, for reasons that will become clear, that improved economic conditions and longer life expectancy will markedly raise the number of people with diabetes beyond the 100 million presently estimated.

WHAT?

The basic problem in diabetes is that the blood sugar is persistently elevated. This may seem a simple point, but a surprising number of patients are unaware of it, particularly those over 65 years of age. Biochemically, a value of 8 mmol/l or more of glucose in a fasting plasma sample is required to satisfy the diagnosis (Chapter 2). For treatment purposes the population of diabetic patients may be split into those who have insulin dependent diabetes (IDDM) and those who are non-insulin dependent (NIDDM). Patients may move from one diagnostic group to the other. Almost 90% of elderly people with diabetes belong to the NIDDM group.

WHY?

In rare cases, blood sugar raised to that diagnostic of diabetes occurs secondarily to conditions such as pancreatic disease, hormonal disturbances (e.g. increased growth hormone in acromegalics), rare genetic disorders, noxious chemicals or, more commonly in the elderly population, stress from intercurrent illnesses such as myocardial infarction or glucose intolerance created by the administration of certain drugs, notably thiazide diuretics and corticosteroids. Usually, however, the cause of diabetes is uncertain, but many have been postulated.

IDDM occurs predominantly in younger people, with a much higher incidence in the winter months, raising the possibility of an association with viral infections in genetically predisposed individuals. Mumps and coxsackie viruses have both been suggested as having a role. This genetic susceptibility is further enhanced by the finding that certain human leucocyte antigens (most notably HLA-DR3 and HLA-DR4) confer up to a fourteenfold risk of acquiring the disease. These antigens are markers on the white blood cells similar to the A, B, O groups on red blood cells. Furthermore, as many as 80% of people with IDDM have circulating islet cell cytoplasmic antibodies, which often are detectable soon after diagnosis and disappear thereafter. Indeed the antibodies may be present 2–7 years prior to the onset of frank diabetes. The term 'type 1' is often used to describe patients who have these antibodies and antigens present, and it is commonly used as a synonym for IDDM. This assocation is not invariable, as some type 1 patients have NIDDM and some patients with IDDM are not type 1. It is simpler to think of patients as requiring insulin or not to keep their blood glucose within physiological limits.

NIDDM is much more common than IDDM, particularly in elderly people. This form of diabetes seems to be inherited, but there are no clear genetic markers as in IDDM. Instead there seem to be a number of factors involved, including heredity and ageing, social class, race and environment.

The risk of developing NIDDM increases steadily with age from the early twenties. It is more common in lower socio-economic groups and in certain racial groups such as the Pima Indians of Arizona, the Tamils of the Indian sub-continent and Jewish people when exposed to the appropriate environmental stimulus. American Negroes are more prone to NIDDM than their white counterparts and some Arab groups also have a high incidence.

The most important environmental factor identified by the World Health Organization is that of obesity. This connection is suggested by the facts that, diabetic patients are on average overweight, glucose tolerance improves with weight loss and obesity is associated with insulin insensitivity. Diets which are high in simple carbohydrates, and physical inactivity have been implicated as possible factors for the increased rates of NIDDM in industrialized societies.

Glucose tolerance declines with age and this can cause problems with the biochemical diagnosis of diabetes (Chapter 2). The decline begins in about the third decade and continues throughout the remainder of adult life. The exact reason is unclear, as glucose absorption from the intestine and insulin production are not greatly altered. It now seems likely, however, that a progressive impairment in the peripheral tissue responsiveness to both insulin and glucose is the explanation. This is witnessed by the fact that most elderly people with NIDDM have raised circulating concentrations of insulin.

Thus it can be appreciated that the causes of NIDDM are truly multifactorial.

2

CLINICAL FEATURES AND CASE DETECTION
Listening, looking and investigating

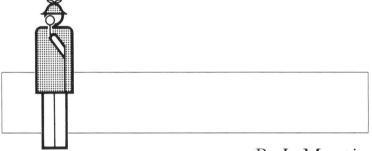

B. J. Martin
and
P. V. Knight

LISTENING AND LOOKING

Although glucose tolerance declines with age, very few elderly people are liable to complain of this to their general practitioner. However, diabetes is common and the increased risk of many debilitating complications, such as blindness and vascular disease, may be mitigated by early diagnosis and adequate care.

There are relatively few elderly people who develop IDDM *de novo*, and in those who do there is often a serious underlying illness. Thus the classical presentation secondary to a raised blood sugar and glycosuria, often seen in younger patients, is much less common. If it occurs the patient will commonly complain of thirst, increased urination, fatigue and weight loss. If the problem goes unrecognized the patient may become acidotic, produce ketones in the blood and urine and eventually slip into coma.

Most elderly diabetic patients have type 2 or NIDDM diabetes. A small number may present with an acute illness related to prolonged hyperglycaemia, which results in very high blood sugars (greater than 50 mmol/l), in turn producing gross dehydration and hypotension and eventually leading to coma (Chapter 10). More commonly elderly people present with increasing thirst, polyuria and some form of skin sepsis, usually fungal, such as pruritus vulvae, to which all diabetic patients are more prone.

Some common symptoms may be wrongly ascribed to old age. These include urinary incontinence arising from the glucose induced polyuria, visual deterioration due to retinopathy or cataract (Chapter 11), foot ulcers (Chapter 8), angina and claudication. These latter complications of diabetes are potentially preventable if the illness is diagnosed early enough.

Thus, it may not be uncommon for the optician to be the first to spot the problem on seeing the haemorrhages and exudates of diabetic retinopathy at a routine eye examination. Similarly, the patient may present to their general practitioner with foot ulcers, often painless, or leg cramps, and the diagnosis of diabetes may be overlooked if not actively considered.

Apart from the obvious findings of complications and the red skin associated with sepsis there may be little external evidence of diabetes in the elderly patient. One sign that can prove useful is the crystallization of urinary sugar onto clothes, shoes or toilet seats that sometimes occurs and may be commented upon by the patient or their spouse.

INVESTIGATING

Many elderly diabetic patients will remain completely asymptomatic and their diagnosis is made only by chance on routine blood or urine testing at a check up for some other condition.

The four principal tests for the detection of 'silent' diabetes are urinary glucose, estimation of random or fasting blood glucose samples, glycosylated haemoglobin (HbA_1), and the glucose tolerance test (GTT).

As many as 50% of elderly individuals with significantly raised blood sugar may have no glycosuria. Thus urine testing is only of use when positive and is of limited application for the monitoring of treatment (Chapter 7).

The use of random blood glucose concentrations can sometimes make the diagnosis of diabetes in elderly people difficult because of the decline in glucose tolerance with age. The post-prandial plasma glucose rises by approximately 0.2 mmol/l per decade and following an oral load one hour values rise by 0.5 mmol/l per decade. Fortunately there is a relatively small age effect on fasting glucose concentrations (0.1 mmol/l per decade) and therefore this is the most stable parameter to measure. A fasting venous sample ≥ 8 mmol/l can be regarded as diabetic.

Only in patients who have equivocal results should a GTT be carried out (Table 2.1). Those patients who are categorized as having impaired glucose tolerance on the basis of this test have a roughly 1 in 10 chance of developing frank diabetes.

Temporary disturbance of glucose metabolism often occurs during acute illnesses, including stroke and myocardial infarction. Drugs such as thiazide diuretics and prednisolone may similarly cause problems. It is uncertain whether this is

Table 2.1 Diagnostic glucose concentrations for 75 g carbohydrate glucose tolerance tests, as defined by the World Health Organization. In the absence of symptoms both fasting and 2 hour blood sugar samples (2HBSS) are required for the diagnosis of diabetes

Diagnosis	Venous whole blood (mmol/l)	Capillary whole blood (mmol/l)	Venous plasma (mmol/l)
Diabetes			
Fasting	>7.0	>7.0	>8.0
2HBSS	>10.0	>11.0	>11.0
Impaired glucose tolerance			
Fasting	<7.0	<7.0	<8.0
2HBSS	>7.0–<10.0	>8.0–<11.0	>8.0–<11.0

temporary, to simply the unmasking of a soon to be manifested latent tendency. Again in cases of doubt a GTT should be carried out once the patient returns to normal health and at least a month after the acute event.

Glycosylated haemoglobin testing has greatly improved the assessment of diabetic control, as it reflects blood glucose concentration over the previous 2–3 months, i.e. the life of a red blood cell. Similarly the test may be used as a screening test and studies have suggested that levels of greater than 10% may be considered diagnostic of diabetes. The patient is not required to fast for this test and it only requires one small sample of blood. However this test is unreliable when the life of the red cell is abnormal, e.g. it gives a falsely reduced result in patients with haemolytic anaemia.

Because of the nature of the assay for glycosylated haemoglobin, the normal range of values varies from laboratory to laboratory, and advice should be sought regarding this locally.

SUMMARY

Listen for the complaints of common geriatric problems such as incontinence and poor vision and don't ascribe them to age.

Look for the possibility of diabetic coma complicating other illnesses. Always consider the possibility of diabetes in patients presenting with skin sepsis, and vascular disease.

Investigating the patient with suspected disease should usually be by means of a fasting blood glucose test, backed up with a glycosylated haemoglobin test and in rare cases a GTT.

3

EDUCATION OF ELDERLY PEOPLE WITH DIABETES

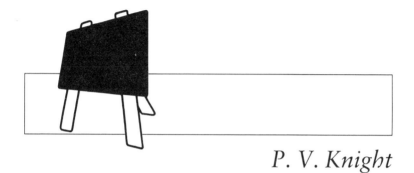

P. V. Knight

In many textbooks of diabetes, education of the patient merits only a paragraph or small chapter tucked away at the end of the main text. However, without knowledge about their condition, patients are unable to motivate themselves towards the attainment of good metabolic control. In addition, several studies have shown conclusively that improved education of people with diabetes decreases their morbidity, and in particular their admission to hospital with hypoglycaemia, hyperglycaemia and foot problems.

Generally the thrust of diabetic education has been towards the younger patient. However, the elderly patient is no less deserving and has a different set of problems to deal with. It should also be remembered that life expectancy at 65 years may be another 15 or 20 years.

IS THERE A PROBLEM IN ELDERLY PATIENTS?

The answer is Yes, there undoubtedly is. Although in the UK many diabetic patients are poorly informed about their condition, elderly people with diabetes, particularly those who are not in need of insulin, are by far the most ignorant. In one survey, the majority of elderly diabetic patients were able to answer an average of less than 20% of a questionnaire on diabetes correctly.

The particular points which seem to confuse elderly patients include the generality of diabetic diet, knowledge of the symptoms of hypoglycaemia and hyperglycaemia, the meaning of urine and blood tests performed at home, awareness of the possibility of complications, and what to do during illness. It would therefore appear that there is considerable scope for improvement in their education.

SPECIFIC PROBLEMS IN EDUCATION OF THE ELDERLY DIABETIC PATIENT

Many elderly patients have little knowledge of how their body functions and often even less desire to gain such expertise.

Therefore, when a diagnosis of diabetes is made the news is often misconstrued in one of two dramatic ways. Either the sufferer feels that diabetes can be shaken off, perhaps with the help of some pills, not unlike a cold, or that they are near to death and would do well to entrust their worldly goods to a next of kin. Between these two poles there are many shades of grey and it is important that the health care team are aware of this problem.

The first task of the educator is to impart what is important and significant, without precipitating undue anxiety.

Sensory deficit

This may take one of four distinct forms or perhaps a combination. Any of these will prove a barrier to the achievement of educational objectives.

First, it is claimed that one third of the population aged over 65 years have a hearing deficit which has 'unfavourable social consequences'. This might be best combated by having a hearing amplification device, such as a 'Contacta' (Appendix C), available to facilitate communication.

Secondly, visual acuity may be decreased, with 20% of elderly men and 18% of women having a corrected visual acuity of 6/18 or less in their better eye. Therefore, this should be actively looked for by the educator; advice on visual aids can be obtained from departments of ophthalmology and the Royal National Institute for the Blind. There is also an age related loss of the ability to differentiate between blue and yellow colour shades. This may have some significance when home glucose monitoring is considered.

Thirdly, tactile sensation is known to diminish with advancing age, and manipulative disability increases, as a consequence of arthritis. Thus, childproof containers for drugs should be avoided and injection aids considered (Chapter 6).

Finally, and perhaps most importantly, approximately 10% of elderly people living at home suffer from a degree of intellectual impairment (usually senile dementia) and in at least half of these the problem is severe. In order to deal with this problem, and the others, if they are severe, it is often necessary to involve the elderly patient's prime carer in the education process.

Multiple pathology, polypharmacy and drug compliance

For many elderly patients, their diabetes may be the least significant disorder in a catalogue of life-long catastrophes. Therefore, realistic treatment and educational objectives must be set for individual patients.

Vast numbers of pharmaceuticals are prescribed for our elderly population. Multiple drug ingestion and the problems of drug interactions are discussed elsewhere (Chapter 9). However, suffice to say that a careful scrutiny must be made for any possible adverse drug reactions, particularly for sulphonylureas and also the exclusion of diabetogenic drugs, such as corticosteroids.

It is often said, tongue in cheek, by many geriatricians that the only thing that saves large numbers of elderly people from significant morbidity is their steadfast refusal to adhere to prescribed drug regimens. It has been estimated that as many as 80% fail to comply, the reasons are multifactorial, but it is my own experience that the probability of compliance is inversely proportional to the number of drugs prescribed. The administration of tablets and perhaps insulin may well be monitored, or carried out by a relative or professional care staff. As in cases of sensory deficit it is just as important to educate the carer as the patient.

Diet

Much will be said about this extremely important topic in the next chapter. Although very few elderly people are actually malnourished many have problems in maintaining a balanced diet.

Perhaps only 30% of elderly patients adhere to a diabetic

diet. This poor compliance is related both to fears that the diet will be expensive, and failure of staff (usually a doctor) to give good advice. Doctors and nurses are notoriously bad about giving appropriate advice (other than an impersonal sheet) on diet. Whilst it is advisable for all carers working regularly with diabetic patients to heighten their knowledge of diabetic dietary instructions, this is often not practical for the generalist. Accordingly, a qualified dietician must see the patient early and often to try to modify dietary regimens to the patient's own particular needs and goals. Patients are unlikely to become hypoglycaemic on diet alone.

Smoking

Many people over the age of 65 years see little point in stopping smoking because 'its done them no harm so far', but smoking greatly increases the risk of peripheral vascular disease well into old age. Thus, it is worthwhile in expending effort on this topic.

Metabolic control

The aim of treatment of diabetes is to ensure as near normal physiological metabolism as possible and hopefully to decrease complications and improve lifestyle. Many physicians, prefer elderly diabetic patients to maintain a little glycosuria, for fear of precipitating hypoglycaemia. However, this will leave the elderly patient open to developing many very disabling complications and often at a faster rate than their younger counterparts.

It has been shown that with proper education and thus, motivation, elderly people can achieve near normoglycaemia without excessive hypoglycaemia. Without this education, the elderly would be greatly at risk. The problem is that it requires a great deal more effort by the educator and patient if good control is to be achieved. All too often the easy route is taken with an exacting penalty being paid by the patient later on.

Good metabolic control is difficult to define numerically as it will depend on individuals. In an elderly person without major physical or mental disability normoglycaemia should be sought vigorously, and is often easier to attain than in younger patients.

WHAT DOES THE PATIENT THINK?

It would be a rash manufacturer that did not employ some market research before releasing a new product to the public. Similarly it is useful to have some idea of how the patient would like to be educated.

There is a hard core of elderly diabetic patients (approximately 37% of insulin dependent diabetics and 16% of non-insulin dependent diabetics) who do not wish further information about their condition. They usually believe that they already have adequate knowledge, which, as we have seen, is quite fallacious. It is a truism that a little knowledge is dangerous, and diabetic clinics must be second only to antenatal clinics in the number of truly horrific stories which are imparted by one patient to another.

The majority of patients, however, do wish to be educated and most would like a book to keep for reference and have this supplemented with one-to-one chats with doctors, dieticians and nurses, as appropriate. Video or film demonstrations are not as popular as with young patients.

HOW TO GO ABOUT IT

When?

Education must start as soon as a reliable diagnosis is made. Often the jump from diagnosis to attainment of good control is never made because education is not pursued.

Where?

In the UK a hospital clinic is still most frequently the first point of contact for many people with diabetes. As the population ages, these clinics will be unable to cope with the ever increasing population of elderly diabetic patients. Indeed many clinics discharge patients at various age bands to concentrate on 'more interesting' younger patients. Shared care of elderly patients between interested general practitioners and hospital specialists may be the best way forward.

Visits to a hospital clinic are normally unstructured in their educational content because of the ever changing medical staff and frequency of visits. In order to derive maximum educational benefit from these visits patients should be enrolled on an educational check list. This list should not only include the topics discussed but also when, by whom, and how well the patient understood them.

This system could run equally well in the general practitioner mini-clinics, such as those in Wolverhampton, and the shared-care systems, such as in Poole and Stirling. The interaction between hospital clinic and community will be explored later (Chapter 14).

Who?

Education of patients is a team effort, with the main members being doctors, nurses and dietitians, who have fairly specific roles to play. Although nurses specially trained in diabetes have come more recently onto the scene, elderly patients often relate more closely with them. They ask them questions that they would not 'bother' the doctor with. The number of highly trained nurse specialists in diabetes is small but they in turn can train others to a degree of proficiency which would allow them to give sound advice in the situations which commonly cause difficulty. Thus district nurses and health visitors might provide a valuable link with the community. It is interesting that educational misconceptions common in patients are also commonly held by nurses and junior doctors.

What?

This is the easiest question to answer, and there is little disagreement over the subject matter patients and carers need to know; these are shown in the list below.

The essentials of diabetic knowledge

1. The nature of diabetes in this patient;
2. The rationale for therapy;
3. The possible complications;
4. Meal and activity planning;
5. The extremes of glycaemia;
6. Coping with illness;
7. How the patient may assess their control;
8. Foot care.

TEACHING AIDS

As yet there is no booklet prepared specifically for elderly diabetic people in Britain, although many hospital departments prepare their own advice sheets. Much of the educational material provided by the British Diabetic Association (BDA) and pharmaceutical companies is excellent, but requires the elderly patient to extrapolate from the experience of younger people. Authors would do well to remember that print should be large and diagrams explicit in such booklets. Computer-assisted learning is inappropriate for the large numbers of patients involved in this age group.

Video presentations may be usefully viewed in a group, but only when skilled advice is at hand to explain any nagging doubts. The videos presently available from the BDA that are applicable to elderly patients are listed below.

Educational videocassettes prepared for the BDA

1. Testing the urine
2. Testing the blood

3. Foot care
4. Diet
5. Type II non-insulin dependent diabetes
6. What is diabetes? (case; general review)
7. Complications of diabetes

SUMMARY

There is no doubt that elderly people with diabetes are much less knowledgeable than their younger counterparts. They are no less in need of instruction, but this needs to be organized on different lines from those presently employed for adolescents. If successful, education of this group will greatly decrease morbidity and improve quality of life.

4

DIETARY ASSESSMENT AND THERAPY

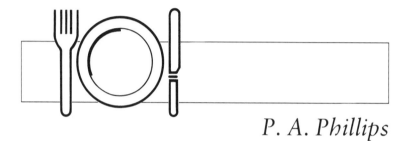

P. A. Phillips

THE ROLE OF DIET

Successful control of diabetes is dependent on dietary management, either alone or in combination with a therapeutic agent.
Recent years have seen alterations to the dietary recom-
mendations for the population as a whole, including reduction
in total calorie intake, and increased fibre and unrefined
carbohydrate diets with reduced fat intake.

The current drive and enthusiasm for this regimen has been
directed towards the more 'youthful' type I insulin dependent
diabetic patient, in an attempt to reduce the incidence of
atheroma and other diabetic complications. This has led,
unfortunately, to less emphasis on dietary treatment for the
elderly diabetic patient. It may be that there is not the urgency
to prevent the onset of diabetic complications (which may
already be present), or there may be doubt over the benefits
which may accrue to these patients from improved long-term
glycaemic control.

However, complacency has no place in the dietary
treatment of diabetes mellitus, whether it be directed to the
type I or type II patient. The task of designing the correct diet
and of eliciting dietary compliance from the elderly patient
should be considered a challenge, particularly when consideration is given to the fact that at least 40% of diabetic
patients are over 60 years of age.

NUTRITION AND AGEING

Ageing is associated with subtle changes in the body, involving
a gradual decline in physiological functions. Carbohydrate
tolerance decreases with age, and this is reflected in the fact
that many elderly patients show elevated random blood
glucose levels.

There is an increased prevalence of poor nutritional intake,
resulting in deficiencies of iron, folate, vitamins B_{12}, C and D.
Thus, elderly people are at risk of developing nutritional
anaemias and bone disorders. Other factors which contribute

to poor nutrient intake include poverty, fear and loneliness. These are all factors which must be considered when assessing and prescribing diets for the elderly patient.

ASSESSMENT OF NORMAL LIFESTYLE

Inappropriate dietary advice is invasive. It can disrupt the routine of the patient, cause needless expense and result in non-compliance.

That dietary compliance is poor is well documented. Care must be taken not to describe the diet as sugar free. This is misleading and results in confusion. A more suitable description is that of a low sugar diet, a term which does not preclude the use of carbohydrate containing foods, such as bread, potatoes, scones etc, so essential in providing a high fibre, high carbohydrate diet.

FAT CONTENT OF THE DIET

The aim in reduction of fat intake is to reduce the incidence of coronary heart disease in diabetic patients. There seems little need to over-restrict the fat content in the diet of the elderly diabetic patient, as this could seriously affect the nutritional quality of the diet. Foods such as margarine and oily fish are important providers of fat, soluble vitamins and, in particular, vitamin D.

Inexpensive protein foods, such as eggs and cheese, have moderate to high fat levels. These should not be over-restricted as this would lead to greater dependence on the more expensive protein foods such as lean red meat and fish. The choice of cheese can be discussed with the patient to suggest low fat levels, but point out that low fat cheese is more expensive than its high fat counterpart. Thus consideration must be given to the patient's financial situation.

Simple guidelines to explain how fat intake can be reduced may be offered along with the diet sheet, for example:

1. Do not fry food (grill or bake instead, where possible);
2. Choose lean varieties of meat and low fat cheeses, where possible;
3. Trim excess fat off meat;
4. Use spreading fats (e.g. butter, margarine) sparingly.

DIABETIC PRODUCTS

These 'alternatives' to preserves and sweets are best avoided by the elderly patient. They are a needless expense and contain sorbitol which can exert an undesirable laxative effect and is high in kilocalories. They are therefore unsuitable for the obese patient. Saccharine and aspartame-based drinks are suitable for all people with diabetes and thus need not be avoided.

THE OBESE DIABETIC PATIENT

Diabetes is exacerbated by obesity. Of those diabetic patients over 65 years of age, the majority are overweight. Weight loss in the elderly diabetic patient is made more difficult by a number of factors which include decreased metabolic rate and decreased mobility.

The achievement of 'average' weight for age and height will, in the elderly diabetic patient, require the imposition of a restriction of 1000–1200 kilocalories.

In those diabetic patients who are housebound and obese, a calorie restriction of 600 kilocalories may be necessary for a short period to establish a definite weight loss. Persuasion, and rehabilitation to improve mobility and well being may be required to encourage compliance.

Frequent, positive, enthusiastic and friendly advice is very important.

General weight reducing advice

1. Avoid sugar and sweet cakes;
2. Avoid fried food. Use butter and margarine sparingly;
3. Have regular meals;
4. Use a sweetener instead of sugar;
5. Cut down on sweet biscuits and white bread. Take whole-meal bread and high fibre foods regularly;
6. Do not use diabetic foods.

The importance of social involvement to the elderly diabetic patient should not be overlooked. It is just as important for the elderly patient, whether obese or not, to have tea and biscuits at a club or friend's house, as it is for a teenager to enjoy a night out with friends. Thus the dietitian will include treats as part of the diet plan to allow for such situations.

Fear and loneliness can affect compliance by producing a general self neglect. The patient becomes apathetic (often aggravated by poor nutrition) and reluctant to prepare meals, losing the ability to prepare meals for themselves through lack of confidence.

Physical disabilities and varying degrees of visual impairment can hinder the preparation of food and force the elderly patient to rely on prepared starchy foods (e.g. pies, pastries, etc) if support services are not available. A diet history taken from the patient should bring these factors to light. An effective diet history will provide such information as the following:

1. Normal meal pattern and timing. From this, intakes of energy, carbohydrate, protein and fat can easily be estimated and any nutritional deficiencies highlighted and corrected;
2. The individual's ability or inability to cook and provide for himself; whether support services (e.g. Meals on Wheels, home helps, etc) are being utilized or will be required;

3. Whether the patient lives alone;
4. The patient's financial situation (e.g. State pension alone or State plus other income source);
5. Physical disabilities (e.g. poor mobility, visual impairment).

On completion of such an assessment, the dietitian can provide dietary advice suitable to the individual's needs. At this stage liaison with other professionals (e.g. occupational therapists, social workers etc) can help alleviate any problems that may occur.

DIABETIC DIETS FOR THE ELDERLY PATIENT

Dietary advice for the elderly patient can range from the simple 'thou shalt not' approach to the full Carbohydrate Exchange System. However, whichever diet system is chosen, emphasis must be on high fibre, low fat foods. Persuading the elderly patient to follow a diet or alter the habits of a lifetime is a challenge. Previously, dietary advice for all people with diabetes was based on a carbohydrate restricted diet (carbohydrate contributing 40% of total energy), allowing a relatively free intake of protein and fat, which tended to result in unrestricted energy intakes.

PRINCIPLES OF DIETARY THERAPY

Recent evidence shows that it is the total energy (kilocalorie) content of the diet and not just carbohydrate restriction which is important in achieving and maintaining glycaemic control in the diabetic.

The energy content of the diet must be related to the individual's requirements, taking into account the patient's age, height, normal activity level and occupation. The carbohydrate content of the diet (from unrefined sources) should supply 50% of the total energy level and there should be a general decrease in fat consumption.

How do these principles relate to the elderly patient?

Many elderly people maintain active lifestyles with high energy requirements, whilst others become increasingly inactive and have low energy requirements. Thus it is undesirable to distribute 'standard' 1200 kilocalorie or 1400 kilocalorie diet sheets without prior assessment of energy needs. Strict calorie control may be difficult to achieve as the elderly diabetic patient may not have the mental agility to estimate both the carbohydrate and kilocalorie content of their food.

CARBOHYDRATES

Traditionally, both simple sugars (sucrose, glucose, etc) and more complex carbohydrates (such as those in wholegrain cereals, peas, beans, etc) were included in the restriction. Thus the elderly diabetic patients tended to rely on the more expensive protein foods (e.g. meat and cheese) for meals and snacks.

Despite advice to the contrary, there remains an anxiety in some not to consume even simple snacks, such as plain biscuits (e.g digestives), for fear they would contribute too much sugar to the diet. Thus advice on carbohydrate sources must be given in a clear simple way to overcome ignorance.

A high fibre diet has been linked to improved glycaemic control; this brings an improved sense of well being to the patient. Foods to be encouraged will therefore include wholemeal bread, cereals, peas, beans, fruit and vegetables. Fibrous foods also have a greater satiety value and may help to reduce the incidence of eating snacks throughout the day. It is unlikely that radical changes to the diet of elderly diabetic patients need to be made, as they are more likely to have 'sensible' meal pattern than the younger patient, who may tend to prefer 'junk food'.

THE ETHNIC GROUP

The broad spectrum of the ethnic population in the UK includes Hindu, Bengali, Moslem, Chinese, Japanese, West Indian

West Indian and African. The main barrier here to compliance and understanding is poor communication.

Dietitians are generally not multi-lingual! They may rely on a member of the patient's family to act as an interpreter. Thus, careful phrasing and questioning must take place during the initial assessment. It is worthwhile seeking an interpreter from a member of their particular community to promote understanding.

It is essential that any dietary advice takes into account the traditional meal pattern and traditional foods, for example chapatis, rice, etc. The dietary advice should preferably be in the patient's own language.

Most elderly ethnic diabetic patients continue to live with their families, a factor which removes the risk of loneliness as a contributor to poor compliance. However, this also presents a problem as meals are prepared for all the family. Therefore fat restriction and calorie restriction for the obese is difficult to achieve without the co-operation of the other members of the family.

Traditional diets tend to be high in fibre, incorporating the use of pulses and legumes (e.g. dhal (lentils) and peas), but where the diet has become 'westernized' chips and sweets cause problems.

SUMMARY OF DIETARY GUIDELINES

The general principles of diabetic dietary therapy for the elderly patient are thus similar to those for younger patients. The diet should be appropriate for the individual's needs; simple sugars should be avoided, and complex carbohydrates (e.g. wholegrain starches, wholemeal bread and cereals) recommended. A general reduction in fat intake would be beneficial for many, but may be difficult to enforce as the elderly patient may rely on inexpensive foods, such as eggs and cheese, which are high in fat, to meet their protein requirements. Handy measures are preferred to the use of scales. If overweight, the weight should be returned to (or close to) the level considered suitable for age and height. Careful motivation and frequent encouragement is essential to improve compliance.

Diets for the immigrant population should not be totally alien to the patient's traditional beliefs and should, where possible, be written in the patient's first language.

Appendix A outlines the basic principles of the diabetic diet suitable for an elderly person. It is essential for the elderly patients to be given more reassurance as finance can be a major worry and care must be taken to ensure that dietary costs will not impede compliance. Inexpensive sources of protein, and the use of fresh fruit and vegetables in season should be emphasized in an attempt to reduce the cost of the diet.

Practical advice about suitable foods which can be stored over winter periods or times of illness must also be given to help prevent a poor nutrient intake at these times.

Total abstinence from alcohol need not be required. A moderate amount of alcohol can be consumed, provided high alcohol products such as 'diabetic beers' are avoided, as those contain a considerable number of kilocalories.

Finally, diet has an important role in the treatment of diabetes. For it to be successful, it is essential to obtain the co-operation of the patient. Education is required at the earliest possible stage and at a time when the patient is relaxed.

5
ORAL THERAPY

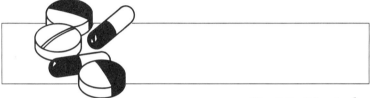

P. V. Knight

Diabetes in the elderly is a common condition. In excess of 80% of elderly diabetic patients will not be receiving insulin and half of them will be prescribed an oral hypoglycaemic agent. Thus, these drugs are in common use and currently the British National Formulary lists 11 such agents (see the list below), although there are another 22 agents available elsewhere. It should be noted that not all of these drugs are available worldwide and, in particular, Metformin is not available in the USA.

Oral hypoglycaemics available in the UK

Sulphonylureas	*Dose range (mg)*
Tolbutamide	500–2000
Chlorpropamide	100–375
Acetohexamide	500–1500
Tolazamide	100–750
Glymidine	500–2000
Glibenclamide	2.5–15
Glipizide	2.5–30
Glibornuride	12.5–75
Gliclazide	40–320
Gliquidone	15–180
Biguanide	
Metformin	500–2000

THE PERFECT DRUG

This would be one that could be taken once a day, lowered the plasma glucose in a physiological manner and did not produce symptomatic hypoglycaemia or other metabolic disruption. Unfortunately, such a drug does not yet exist.

There tend to be two attitudes to starting oral therapy for diabetes in the elderly. The first is that it really doesn't matter and elderly patients do not require treatment unless blood glucose is sky high (i.e. >22 mmol/l). As previously intimated (Chapter 3) this is foolish. The second, but no less illogical theory, is that we would be better to commence oral therapy immediately, as the elderly 'never' comply with diets.

It is my practice only to commence oral anti-diabetic therapy (in the non-emergency situation) when the post-prandial plasma glucose remains elevated, in excess of 12 mmol/l following one month of adequate dietary therapy, as outlined in Chapter 4. The plasma glucose value is one of individual preference which may be disputed. It should always be stressed, however, that tablets are an adjunct to dietary therapy, not a substitute.

CHOOSING THE CORRECT DRUG

Sulphonylureas

This group provides 10 of the 11 oral hypoglycaemics available in the UK. Their potency depends largely on the extent to which they are inactivated by liver metabolism and their method of excretion, i.e. via the biliary or renal system.

How these drugs work is unclear. It is generally thought that in the short term sulphonylureas stimulate insulin secretion. However, in the longer term this is not the case and their hypoglycaemic action appears to be related to a reduction of liver glucose production and some enhancement of insulin effect due to action around the insulin receptors.

Symptomatic hypoglycaemia, which can occur with any of these preparations, is not really a side effect but an extension of their pharmacological action. It is their main drawback and usually occurs for one of three reasons:

1. The dose of drug is excessive in relation to the degree of hyperglycaemia, and the patients renal and hepatic function;
2. The patient may eat inadequately and miss meals. This is a particular problem in unsupervised elderly patients with moderate degrees of intellectual impairment;
3. All sulphonylureas are highly bound to proteins which circulate in the blood. This is particularly true of the

so-called 'first generation' agents, e.g. acetohexamide, chlorpropamide, tolbutamide and tolazamide. The sulphonyl urea may be displaced from these proteins by concomitant administration of drugs such as aspirin and warfarin as they have a greater affinity for the proteins. This will give more 'free' drug available for action, and so enhance their hypoglycaemic effect.

Therefore, in an elderly population who may eat irregularly and have significantly diminished renal function, the logical choice of drug should be one that has a short half-life, is excreted by the liver or, if excreted by the kidney, has largely inactive metabolites. Drugs included in this category are tolbutamide, glipizide and gliquidone. However, all of these can produce symptomatic hypoglycaemia, although the first and only case of gliquidone associated hypoglycaemia was reported recently.

The choice of agent is largely a personal one, but it is my practice to avoid chlorpropamide in the elderly patient because of its markedly prolonged half-life. This may lead to nocturnal hypoglycaemia, which could be fatal. It should also be remembered that a single dose of a short acting agent may be sufficient to produce physiological blood glucose concentrations in the elderly patient over a period of 24 hours.

Drug failures

It should be remembered that sulphonyl ureas are not effective in all patients, and neither can they be guaranteed to be efficacious for ever.

Approximately 10–20% of patients, even if they are properly selected, will fail to respond to sulphonylurea treatment from the onset. These so-called 'primary failures' tend to have weight loss and have grossly uncontrolled diabetes mellitus which requires insulin therapy. The reasons for this phenomenon are unclear.

Following initial response to therapy there is another group of patients who have a 'secondary failure' to sulphonylureas.

This may occur for clear reasons, such as intercurrent illness or failure to adhere to diet. This group often respond once more when the obstacle has been removed. However, there is another group of secondary failures in whom there is no clear reason for the event. This may be expected to occur in approximately 5–10% of patients per year. Occasionally patients may respond to one sulphonylurea when they have failed on another.

Thus, one cannot prescribe sulphonylureas and forget about them. These agents must be monitored because of their tendency to have diminished efficacy with time and conversely their risk of producing acute hypoglycaemia.

Biguanides

These drugs are unavailable in the USA and presently Metformin is the only one prescribable in the UK. This drug can be used alone or in combination with any of the sulphonylurea agents and it has theoretical advantages in the elderly patient in that it does not produce symptomatic hypoglycaemia and has useful weight reducing effects.

There are three main theories of the mechanism of action of Metformin. First, inhibition of intestinal glucose absorption; secondly, increased peripheral utilization of glucose, and thirdly inhibition of hepatic glucose production.

Metformin's occasionally fatal flaw is that it disrupts intermediary metabolism and can produce lactic acidosis which has a high mortality rate. Lactic acidosis is more likely in anoxia and when liver detoxification and renal excretion are reduced. It has been suggested that Metformin should be avoided in all cases of cardiac, respiratory, renal and hepatic impairment. This has led to random age barriers for the prescription of Metformin being suggested, because of the increased incidence of these disorders with increasing age. This, in my view, is a little illogical as some patients aged 80 years may have none of these problems while others aged 50 years may have all of them.

Therefore, each individual should be assessed separately.

Metformin should be avoided in patients with (or with a recent history of) overt cardiac, renal, respiratory or hepatic failure. Provided biochemical values are within normal limits for the elderly patient there does not appear to be an increased risk in those aged over 65 years.

There was not a single case of Metformin induced lactic acidosis reported in the UK from 1972–1982.

Guar gum

Guar is not strictly speaking a drug. It is a non-absorbable carbohydrate which is commonly used in food technology as a thickening agent. Several studies have shown that it may lower post-prandial blood glucose, although this remains controversial. The situation in the elderly patient is unclear. One study showed that administration helped weight loss but did not significantly lower blood glucose.

SUMMARY

Oral hypoglycaemic agents have a definite role to play in the management of elderly diabetic patients. The patients must be selected carefully and oral therapy should not be considered as a substitute for adherence to dietary regimens. Careful follow-up of the patient is required to assess efficacy and side effects.

Following patient selection I find it best to start with a short acting sulphonylurea such as gliquidone, particularly if the patient is near normal weight. If this approach is unsuccessful, or if the patient is markedly obese from the outset, I will often add metformin or prescribe this alone, provided all the exclusion criteria have been strictly observed.

The choice of oral hypoglycaemic agent should be based on firm pharmacological principles, but often remains rather personal. It is a good idea, as with beta-blockers and sedatives, to get to know a few agents thoroughly rather than trying the field.

6

INSULIN THERAPY

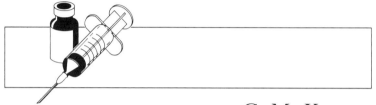

C. M. Kesson

Insulin is a major regulator of overall metabolism, having important effects on fat and protein metabolism in addition to its action on carbohydrates. The increase in insulin secretion which accompanies food ingestion facilitates the storage of all the ingested nutrients, and the fall in insulin level which normally occurs in between meals enhances the mobilization and production of metabolic fuels. In addition insulin is a hormone associated with regulation of the blood glucose concentration. As a major aim of treatment in diabetes is to establish metabolic control, maintaining blood glucose levels within limits and avoiding either hyperglycaemia or hypoglycaemia, it is necessary to supply the correct dose of insulin. While a great many advances have been made since the discovery of insulin at the University of Toronto in 1921, the fact remains that insulin is a polypeptide hormone of complex structure which is destroyed by gastric juices and has, therefore, to be injected rather than ingested orally.

INSULIN SOURCES

Insulin preparations, used in treatment of diabetic patients, can be obtained in three ways.

1. From bovine pancreas glands – 'beef insulin'
2. From porcine pancreas glands – 'pork insulin'
3. Manufactured by recombinant DNA technology – 'human insulin'

The insulin obtained from animal sources is purified by crystallization but the product is not identical to human insulin.

Pork insulin differs from human insulin by only one amino acid, but beef insulin has three amino acids different from human insulin. The beef preparations are slightly more antigenic and, if insulin from an animal source is used, the pork variety is to be preferred.

TYPES OF INSULIN

Insulin preparations, which currently number around 40 in the British National Formulary, can be classified according to duration of action, into fast acting, intermediate acting or long acting preparations. Some examples of these are listed below.

Insulin preparations

Short acting
Human type – Human Actrapid, Human Velosulin, Humulin S
Pork type   – Velosulin
Beef type   – Hypurin Neutral, Quicksol

Intermediate acting
Human type – Humulin I, Human Initard, Human Mixtard, Humulin M1, Humulin M2, M3, M4
Pork type   – Initard, Mixtard
Beef type   – Isophane Insulin, Hypurin Isophane

Long acting
Human type – Human Monotard, Human Ultratard, Human Protaphane, Human Insulatard, Humulin ZN
Pork type   – Insulatard
Beef type   – Hypurin Lente, Tempulin, Hypurin Protamine Zinc

WHEN DO DIABETIC PATIENTS NEED INSULIN?

All patients with type 1 diabetes require insulin every day. This is usually given by subcutaneous injection, but patients with type 2 diabetes, who are normally controlled with diet alone or with diet and oral hypoglycaemic drugs, may require insulin on some occasions, for example during acute infections, following major trauma or during major surgery. Following tablet treatment for some years, if the pancreas is exhausted and no longer responds to oral hypoglycaemic drugs, then type

2 patients require to change treatment to daily insulin injections.

WHICH INSULIN PREPARATION SHOULD BE USED?

A number of considerations have to be taken into account before selecting the appropriate method of insulin therapy. Because of increasing evidence that strict metabolic control is important in prevention of the long term complications of diabetes it is vital to try to control the blood glucose level throughout the 24 hours. With subcutaneous injection of insulin, this can best be achieved by giving once daily a single injection of a long acting insulin and, in addition, giving an injection of fast acting insulin perhaps three times daily before each meal. However, some patients are unable or unwilling to inject insulin four times daily and many patients are treated with intermediate acting insulin injections twice daily. In older patients, where there is less worry about long term sequelae of diabetes, it may be reasonable to control diabetes and render the patient asymptomatic by giving them a once daily injection of a long acting insulin. While a once daily insulin injection will not achieve the best possible glycaemic control throughout the 24 hours, it can often suffice to allow the patient freedom from symptoms, and indeed would perhaps be the treatment of choice for those patients who are unable to inject their own insulin, relying on assistance from nurses or relatives to inject their daily insulin.

INSULIN DOSE

It is impossible to state what dose of insulin a patient will require before insulin treatment is started. On average, most patients will require between 30 and 60 units of insulin daily, but it is often useful to begin with a small dose of fast acting insulin, perhaps 8 units twice daily before meals and increase the dose as required with respect to blood glucose levels. Once a daily requirement is established this may not vary much in elderly patients, whereas younger patients may have considerable variations in insulin requirement with respect to variations in energy expenditure. The elderly patient is often able to be satisfactorily controlled without recourse to daily variation in insulin dose.

INSULIN INJECTION

Insulin is usually given by subcutaneous injection and it is important that all patients are assessed to ensure that they can manage to inject the prescribed dose of insulin. Disabilities, unrelated to diabetes, such as marked tremor or poor vision, can preclude the patient from satisfactory self-management of insulin injections and for these patients an insulin injection device, such as a pen injector, may be a worthwhile alternative to the conventional syringe.

Various injection devices are now available and it is likely that many more will be marketed in the near future. Most now hold cartridges of insulin and so eliminate the necessity to load a syringe from a vial of insulin. The injection dosage is delivered subcutaneously through a fine needle. Needleless insulin injectors are also available but must still be loaded from insulin vials and have the advantage of not using a needle to penetrate the skin. The high cost of this sort of device will ensure that widespread use will not occur.

PROBLEMS WITH THE USE OF INSULIN

Hypoglycaemia

Hypoglycaemia is, by far and away, the most important acute complication of insulin therapy and is dealt with in Chapter 10. It is of great importance that all patients who require insulin treatment should carry with them, wherever they are, about 30 g of carbohydrate in the form of glucose or sweets so that they can, themselves, treat the initial symptoms of hypoglycaemia.

Insulin absorption

After injection, absorption of insulin is affected by blood flow and an increase in blood flow will increase the absorption rate. Increased exercise in the injected limb or increased ambient temperature, for example, following a hot bath or sunbathing, can increase the absorption rate of insulin. There is also some anatomical variation, in that insulin injected into the abdominal region is absorbed more quickly than that injected into the lower limbs.

Lipohypertrophy

If insulin is injected repeatedly into the same small area, it can often produce fibrous, fatty tumours which are unsightly and can cause problems with delayed absorption from such tissues. It is simple to prevent this complication by rotating insulin injection sites.

Lipoatrophy

This complication is now seen infrequently as it is thought to be an allergic response to poorly purified insulin preparations and is not associated with the highly purified pork or human insulin preparations which are now available.

Insulin allergy

Systemic allergy may occur at any time during insulin treatment with an urticarial eruption which may lead to anaphylactic shock. However, insulin allergy is extremely uncommon and, on the very rare occasions it does occur, it can be treated by desensitizing the patients with small and gradually increasing doses of highly purified pork or human insulin.

7

MONITORING CONTROL OF DIABETES IN THE ELDERLY PATIENT

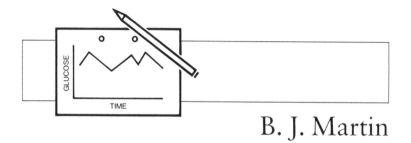

B. J. Martin

WHOSE RESPONSIBILITY?

The answer to this question depends, to a large extent, on local circumstances, however, it is imperative that all diabetic patients are seen for review from time to time.

In the past, in Britain, the follow-up of diabetic patients was mainly conducted at hospital clinics and, at the present time, many patients continue to rely on the hospital service; however, in recent years there has been some movement towards community care with an expansion in the establishment of general practitioner based mini-clinics and more frequent utilization of specialized trained diabetic health visitors and district liaison nursing sisters (Chapters 13 and 14). These changes are particularly suited to elderly patients, who may find attendance at their own general practitioner less inhibiting and more convenient than hospital clinic visits.

PATIENT CARE

Whether supervision of control is hospital or community based it is important that the requirements of the elderly diabetic patient are met. The popular misconception that, due to infirmity and diminished intellectual reserve, the ageing patient is unwilling or incapable of making minor changes in lifestyle or learning simple techniques which could improve the quality of diabetic control should be corrected. Similarly, perhaps because most elderly diabetic patients are non-insulin dependent and are often asymptomatic, good control could be thought to be less important and education unnecessary. This view is erroneous since there is a high prevalence of complications in elderly diabetics and increasingly evidence accumulates that much of the resulting chronic debility can be prevented by institution of adequate control which should be achieved through satisfactory education of the patient.

Most elderly diabetic patients remain independent, with well preserved intellectual function, and their requirements do not differ greatly from those of younger patients. Given appropriate educational opportunities they are capable of participating in the day to day monitoring of diabetic control at home and can be supervised locally with referral to specialist centres only for specific problems.

HOME MONITORING

Essentially there are three options:

1. No monitoring;
2. Urine testing;
3. Blood testing.

The evidence in favour of the benefit of good diabetic control is such that, where at all possible, some form of monitoring should be undertaken. Urine testing for glucose is simple to perform and can certainly alert the patient to potential danger due to hyperglycaemia. Urine testing for glycosuria is not really satisfactory if the aim is to establish metabolic control because the renal threshold for glucose rises with age and thereby a negative test for glycosuria can occur simultaneously with a degree of hyperglycaemia. Urine testing for glycosuria is of no value for warning of hypoglycaemia. In addition, some people have low renal thresholds for glucose and will have frequent positive urine tests for glycosuria although their blood glucose level is satisfactory.

Urine testing for proteinuria, on the other hand, is a valuable screening test for evidence of incipient renal problems, but this could be carried out at intermittent review and it is not necessary for the patient to check frequently for protein in urine. Testing for ketonuria can be valuable when hyperglycaemia is present but is certainly not an essential test for an elderly patient to carry out routinely.

Home blood glucose monitoring has well documented advantages over urine testing in day to day assessment of diabetic control. The technique is now widely employed in young insulin dependent diabetic patients but, until recently, was considered impractical and unnecessary in the elderly. Experience now shows us that a significant number of elderly diabetic patients adapt well to the introduction of home blood glucose monitoring and prefer it to urine testing, which some find distasteful. The technique is particularly useful in the elderly insulin dependent diabetic patient, where the renal threshold for glucose may be high, but it can also be employed beneficially in those patients who do not require insulin. The technique can be modified to suit the capabilities and needs of the individual. Thus, with appropriate instruction, the small minority of highly motivated elderly insulin dependent diabetic patients can learn to adjust their own insulin dose in respect to their blood glucose recording. More commonly the patients may check their blood glucose level on a number of occasions and produce some evidence to assist their attendant in interpreting their diabetic control and aid in rational therapeutic changes.

Where appropriate, a relative or carer may perform blood glucose sampling and recording. The frequency of blood sampling depends on the needs of the individual, for example some brittle insulin dependent patients may require daily blood glucose monitoring, whilst a glucose profile (3 or 4 samples checked in one day) once a week or once a month may suffice for more stable, non-insulin dependent patients. Frequent blood glucose profiles can be used to assess drug therapy in non-insulin dependent patients receiving oral hypoglycaemic therapy. Combined with symptom diaries to record episodes of suspected minor hypoglycaemia, the technique may be invaluable in excluding nocturnal hypoglycaemia, a potential, and often neglected, problem in elderly patients taking oral hypoglycaemic drugs. When adequate and safe control is achieved the frequency of recording can be reduced to the minimum. Recent experience has shown that the rate of successful blood sampling is very high when home monitoring is introduced, at least in selected elderly patients, and can lead to improvement in diabetic control. Employment of the technique contributes to better understanding of the relationship between food and blood glucose and provides valuable information for both physician and patient.

LONG TERM CONTROL

Whereas home blood glucose monitoring and, to a much lesser extent, urine testing for glycosuria are helpful in day to day diabetic control, the measurement of glycosylated haemoglobin permits assessment of control over a much longer period, usually thought to be the preceding 4–8 weeks. In simple terms, when the red cells circulate in the bloodstream, glucose attaches to the haemoglobin within the red cell. In people who do not have diabetes, less than 9% of the haemoglobin has this glucose attached or is glycosylated (n.b. laboratory reference ranges vary). The reaction of glycosylation depends only on the length of time the red cells circulate and the concentration of blood glucose. If there is no haematological problem and the red cells circulate for the normal time, then the percentage of haemoglobin glycosylated gives an indication of the blood glucose level. Thus, if diabetic control has been poor and blood levels have been too high the glycosylated haemoglobin value will be raised above the upper limit. The amount by which this value is raised above the upper limit will depend on how high the blood glucose levels have been, so the glycosylated haemoglobin is a good test to use intermittently to assess diabetic control.

SCREENING FOR COMPLICATIONS

As with all patients who have diabetes, it is useful to screen for early evidence of any of the well known complications; therefore, ophthalmic examination, test of renal function, examination of feet and so forth should be carried out regularly.

To sum up, monitoring of diabetes is important. Monitoring of metabolic control and institution of satisfactory control leads to a better quality of life. Early detection of a complication will enable the institution of appropriate treatment at the earliest stage and can be of great value.

8
FOOT CARE

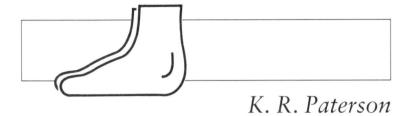

K. R. Paterson

FOOT PROBLEMS AND CHIROPODY

Few other aspects of the management of the diabetic patient are so amenable to careful prevention and treatment than foot problems, and yet few aspects of diabetic management are so frequently ignored, often with disastrous consequences for the patient. Major foot lesions, sometimes requiring surgical intervention and even amputation, can arise from trivial initial damage which is left untreated or is managed inappropriately.

THE NATURE OF THE PROBLEM

Foot problems fall into four broad categories:

1. Common lesions also occurring in non-diabetics (e.g. corns);
2. Foot ulceration (the main challenge to diabetic footcare);
3. Ischaemia and gangrene (diabetic patients are at particular risk);
4. Infection (often as a result of minor trauma).

THE AETIOLOGY OF THE PROBLEM

Foot problems in diabetes are not due to any abnormality specific to the feet, but represent an interaction of diabetic neuropathy and peripheral vascular disease as predisposing factors in the diabetic population, with environmental factors or other medical problems acting as the precipitants in individual patients. The type of foot lesion seen in any one patient depends on the outcome of this interaction. Predisposing factors are outlined below:

1. Diabetic neuropathy (Chapter 11)
   (a) Motor neuropathy leading to abnormal foot shape and stress on toes and the balls of the feet.

(b) Sensory neuropathy leading to loss of various aspects of sensation, such that minor trauma may go unnoticed and the severity of major injury underestimated.

(c) Autonomic neuropathy, by alteration of blood flow in the foot, may further predispose to ulceration and delay healing.

2. Peripheral vascular disease
There is evidence that this is more common in diabetic patients (particularly smokers), especially below the knee where calcification frequently affects the small vessels of the foot as well as the major arteries.

3. Impaired resistance to infection
Both cellular and blood borne methods of combating infection have been shown to be impaired in poorly controlled diabetes, though good metabolic control improves matters. This compounds a situation which already exists in the elderly population as a whole.

PRECIPITATING FACTORS

Whilst many diabetic patients are severely affected by these predisposing factors for foot problems, the development of a foot lesion usually requires an external precipitant, such as:

1. Mechanical trauma from ill-fitting shoes, perhaps compounded by neuropathy or distortion of the foot by oedema;

2. Heat trauma often due to the over-zealous warming of feet with poor circulation by hot water bottles etc;

3. Chemical trauma from external agents available over the counter to treat corns and callouses etc. The elderly skin is fragile and do-it-yourself chiropody of even simple lesions should be actively discouraged.

MANAGEMENT OF FOOT PROBLEMS

Management of foot problems in diabetic patients can be considered under three headings:

1. Prevention of foot problems;
2. Recognition and management of minor problems;
3. Recognition and management of major problems.

1. Prevention

Prevention of diabetic foot problems must be a part of the education of the diabetic patient and should be reinforced whenever and wherever the patient is being reviewed. In addition, though foot inspection forms part of the complications review of all diabetic patients, it is essential that the patient undertakes regular care and inspection of his or her own feet in order that any damage which does occur can be detected and treated as early as possible. Simple advice, preferably written, should be given to each patient and should include:

1. Daily washing of the feet – the feet should be washed every day in soapy water (no antiseptic is necessary), well rinsed and then dried carefully, paying special attention to the clefts between the toes;
2. Inspection of the feet – after washing, the feet should be closely inspected looking for any redness or blistering (evidence of friction) and any cracks, cuts or punctures. Patients should be told that their feet may be slightly numb and that inspection must substitute for the feeling which they lack;
3. Shoes – comfortable shoes of the correct size (neither too tight nor so large as to permit excessive movement of the feet) are essential. High heeled shoes which cause excessive pressure on the toes must be avoided. New shoes should be 'broken-in' carefully, wearing the shoe for an increasing length of time on each occasion and checking the feet carefully after each wearing;
4. Socks – socks, especially cotton socks, protect the feet from frictional damage when walking much more efficiently than nylon stockings or tights. Bare feet, either in shoes or on open floors, are very risky as injuries can easily occur;

5. Toenails – simple cutting of the toenails can be undertaken by the patient if eyesight is satisfactory and the toes can be reached without too much difficulty. The nails should be cut straight across, removing any sharp corners but avoiding cutting down the sides of the nail. If vision is poor or the patient has problems reaching the foot or working with scissors or nail-clippers then a chiropodist should undertake toenail cutting on a regular basis;

6. Foot care – all other foot care, with the exception of simple padding around corns and callouses, should be undertaken by a chiropodist or nurse. The use of corn and wart salves and corn plasters should be proscribed, as should be the cutting of corns;

7. Damage limitation – any foot abnormality, however minor, should immediately be brought to the attention of the doctor, nurse or chiropodist in order that any necessary treatment can be instituted as early as possible.

These simple rules, if followed closely, would remove many of the precipitants of foot lesions and could prevent most of the foot problems which occur in diabetic patients. To the elderly patient, faced with changes in diet and medication at the diagnosis of diabetes, foot problems may seem very trivial and therefore the importance of these rules must be reiterated regularly. In addition, the adverse effects of cigarette smoking on the peripheral circulation must be emphasized and the patient encouraged to reduce or stop smoking.

2. Minor foot problems

A minor foot problem can be defined as a single non-penetrating lesion in a foot which shows no evidence of significant ischaemia, no major spreading infection (e.g. cellulitis) and with no deformity or previous surgery. Such problems are usually amenable to simple, relatively non-invasive out-patient treatment and are often managed by doctors, nurses and chiropodists in the community. Before a lesion can be classed as minor it is essential that adequate clinical examination of the foot and leg is undertaken to assess the extent of peripheral vascular disease and neuropathy. If necessary, X-rays must be obtained to ensure that the superficial lesion is not contiguous with deeper damage (e.g. osteomyelitis beneath a heel ulcer).

FOOT ULCERS

The typical diabetic foot ulcer occurs in an area of abnormal pressure on the foot and often starts, therefore, on an area of thickened skin or callous. Initially the area may appear bruised, due to oozing of blood below the thickened skin, but later the thickened skin will be shed (or can be cut away) to reveal the flat, reddish/pink early granulation tissue which has developed on the base of the ulcer. Typically there is no pain; if the patient presents before the callous skin has been broken then there is little infection but if the granulation tissue has been exposed for some time then infection is common.

Initial management involves careful removal of the callous skin and hyperkeratosis around the ulcer to leave the ulcer base surrounded by 'normal' skin. If the ulcer is clean then it should simply be irrigated with saline or hypochlorite solution and a dry non-stick dressing applied. After obtaining a swab for bacteriological culture, a similar approach may be adequate for minor infections but if there is major infection with slough then careful use of wound cleaning agents such as 'Debrisan' or 'Milton 1 : 4' may be helpful. Chemical cleansing agents, especially those containing irritants such as salicylic acid, are best avoided.

Any 'flare' around the ulcer suggesting soft tissue infection should be treated with systemic antibiotics. Most infections are due to *Staphylococcus aureus*, though frequently more than one organism is found on swabbing the ulcer and streptococci and anaerobic bacteria may be involved. Initial treatment is usually with an anti-staphylococcal antibiotic such as flucloxacillin (1–2 g/d) or fusidic acid (1.5 g/d). If the ulcer seems ischaemic or very malodorous then anaerobes may also be present and metronidazole (1.2 g/d) should be added.

The antibiotic treatment may need to be modified in the light of the culture and sensitivity report on the initial swab. Treatment should continue until all evidence of spreading local infection has gone, usually 7–10 days, but need not be continued until healing has occurred.

With adequate local cleaning, treatment of infection and regular dressing, usually daily, most ulcers will begin to heal. However, full healing of the ulcer can only be achieved if the abnormal local pressure which produced the ulcer is removed. If the ulcer is not on a weight-bearing area, local padding and minor modification of shoes may be sufficient but this aim may be very difficult to achieve with ulcers occurring on the sole of the foot, as normal walking will apply unacceptable pressure. A total ban on walking might appear ideal but is rarely possible, even in hospital, and can produce serious long-term loss of mobility in elderly patients. All patients should be asked to limit their walking as much as possible but additional measures to relieve pressure are usually taken.

1. Local padding – padding over the ulcer, either with gauze or foam, may ease local pressure a little but may also, however, cause the patient to apply unusual loads on other parts of the foot and risk the development of further ulcers. Local padding may be very useful in view of its simplicity but it must be used with caution.
2. Insoles – custom-made insoles can be formed from firm foam or Plastazote, the insole spreading loads evenly over the whole sole with the exception of the area of the ulcer, where a hole in the insole reduces the load. They are very effective in promoting ulcer healing, though care must be taken to ensure that they are only used in shoes which are sufficiently large, as chafing may occur.
3. Surgical shoes – expensive, unsightly and often heavy, surgical shoes are rarely required for the patient with only a minor foot lesion, though they are obviously useful if there is significant foot deformity. Lightweight 'comfort' shoes may be useful in some patients, being cheaper and easier to make and also less of a limitation on mobility.
4. Plaster casts – encasing the lower leg and foot in a

close-fitting plaster cast avoids friction, spread loads very evenly over the whole foot and leg and, with the provision of a walking heel, permits walking. The treatment may be very effective but the cast has to be very carefully applied to avoid producing its own pressure or friction lesions and, in the elderly, may significantly limit mobility and thus remove one of its main advantages.

Prolonged careful dressing of an ulcer, with sustained efforts to reduce pressure and friction at the ulcer site, will usually lead to ulcer healing, though the time required may be several months in the case of large ulcers. Once healing has occurred, the close attention which led to healing must be maintained as the new skin is initially very thin and fragile and will rapidly ulcerate if exposed to excessive pressure. Indeed healing of an ulcer is the best time to begin secondary preventive measures, designed to prevent further problems in what is obviously a vulnerable foot. Education should be reinforced and consideration given to whether insoles or similar preventive appliances should be used in the longer term. Full mobilization should be achieved gradually over several weeks and care should be taken to minimize stresses on the healed foot over this time. Regular review, preferably by a trained chiropodist, should be undertaken on all patients who have ever had a foot ulcer.

Other minor problems include ingrown toenails, corns, callouses and plantar warts. In the elderly diabetic patient these should all be carefully assessed by a practitioner with experience in dealing with them.

3. Major foot problems

Major foot problems encompass the spectrum of lesions which occur singly or multiply in a foot which has evidence of significant ischaemia, deformity (either due to neuropathy or previous amputation), penetration (e.g. into underlying bone) or spreading infection. Any of these features can lead to rapid

progression of the lesion to a stage at which surgical intervention may be required and therefore such problems need to be
identified early and managed vigorously, often with specialist
help. Full consideration of the management of these problems
is outwith the scope of this book.

CONCLUSIONS

Diabetic foot problems are common, usually readily preventable and often easily treated in the early stages, but are also
potentially serious and can lead to permanent loss of independence and mobility in otherwise reasonably fit elderly people.
Constant vigilance by all involved in the management of
diabetes, including the patient, paramedical and nursing staff
and the doctor, is essential if disability is to be avoided.

9

GENERAL PRESCRIBING PROBLEMS IN ELDERLY DIABETIC PATIENTS

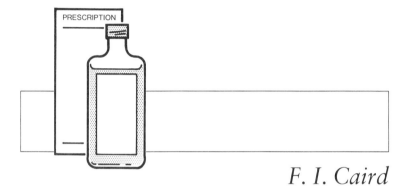

F. I. Caird

The same general principles apply to prescribing for elderly diabetic patients as for non-diabetic patients. In the great majority of instances the prescription of drugs and adverse reactions to them are no different, but there are a number of particular problems. The difficulties that elderly patients have with compliance with drug therapy are perhaps somewhat greater in the elderly diabetic patients, who may have to take medication for diabetes in addition to that for other conditions. There is thus an inevitable tendency towards multiple drug therapy, which is one of the main contributory factors both to the occurrence of adverse drug reactions and to the patient's difficulty with compliance. Other common causes of the latter include poor vision (to which diabetic eye problems may contribute), poor manipulative skills in the hands, and, most important of all, intellectual impairment.

It follows from these general considerations that, with the exceptions detailed below, there should be no hesitation in prescribing non-diabetic drugs to diabetic patients, with the further proviso that the number of drugs that an individual patient is required to take at any one time is not large, preferably not more than three.

The principal problems in prescribing for elderly patients are (1) diabetogenic drugs, (2) drugs which may mask the signs of hypoglycaemia and thus potentiate it, (3) interactions between a variety of drugs and sulphonylureas, (4) particular adverse effects to which the elderly diabetic patient may be prone because of the specific complications of diabetes, and (5) proprietary preparations that contain sugar.

DRUGS THAT INCREASE BLOOD GLUCOSE

The principal diabetogenic drugs are the corticosteroids and the thiazide diuretics. The effects of the former are dose dependent, and glucose tolerance may be substantially impaired by large doses, both in diabetic patients on dietary therapy alone, and also, perhaps to a lesser extent, in those on hypoglycaemic drugs. The effects may occur either soon after the initiation of corticosteroid therapy, i.e. within a few days, or may take much longer to appear; increased blood glucose levels and the appearance of diabetic symptoms are the main manifestations.

The second large class of diabetogenic drugs are the thiazide diuretics. Their diabetogenic action results from impairment of the response of the islet cells to raised blood glucose levels, and it may be potentiated by the potassium deficiency which the thiazides themselves may produce. The diabetogenic effect is, for practical purposes, only seen in diabetic patients on dietary therapy alone, and may take many months to develop. If thiazides need to be continued, and cannot be replaced by substantially less diabetogenic diuretics such as frusemide, the hyperglycaemia may be relatively easily managed by the addition of small doses of a sulphonylurea.

DRUGS THAT MASK HYPOGLYCAEMIA

The large class of beta-adrenergic blocking drugs have as their principal adverse effect in diabetics the masking of the peripheral sympathetic manifestations of hypoglycaemia, such as sweating and tachycardia. The patient may therefore not recognize early hypoglycaemia, and its neurological effects may thus be unexpected. This adverse reaction to beta-blockers usually only affects patients on hypoglycaemic agents, such as sulphonylureas or insulin, since those on dietary therapy very rarely become hypoglycaemic. There is thus little reason whatever to deny them the benefits of beta-blockers given, for instance, for hypertension. Beta-blockers may aggravate the symptoms of peripheral vascular disease, to which diabetic patients are prone, and should therefore not be given to those with this complication.

INTERACTION WITH SULPHONYLUREAS

Sulphinpyrazone and sulphamethoxazole both inhibit sulpho-nylurea metabolism, and the effects of the latter drugs may therefore be increased by this combination. A similar inhibition of glipizide metabolism has been described with cimetidine, and similar precautions are therefore necessary in this instance. In all three cases, it is wise to halve the dose of sulphonylureas in the first instance if any of these interacting drugs need to be given.

PROBLEMS BECAUSE OF COMPLICATIONS

The problem with prescribing for elderly diabetic patients is that of reactions between a variety of drugs and the complications of diabetes. That concerning peripheral vascular disease and beta-blockers has already been mentioned. The particular complication and the particular drugs which give rise to virtually all the problems in this area are diabetic neuropathy and antihypertensive drugs of all types. The combination may result in increase in postural blood pressure drop and in symptomatic postural hypotension. This side effect can, however, be looked for, and guarded against, by recording the blood pressure in both lying and standing positions, as should be done with all hypotensive drugs in all patients.

PROPRIETARY DRUGS

Sugar-containing proprietary medicines (e.g. cough medicines) are probably best avoided by diabetic patients, but are unlikely to do much harm over a short period.

10
HYPERGLYCAEMIA AND HYPOGLYCAEMIA

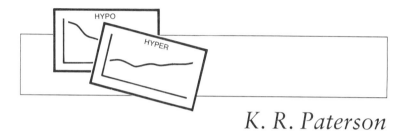

K. R. Paterson

Marked abnormalities of the blood glucose are usually seen at the diagnosis of diabetes but normal values can be returned to and plasma glucose maintained at reasonably acceptable levels with treatment. In the course of management, changes in the disease itself and changes in the general health of the patient may lead to significant variations in blood glucose control which require specific intervention. This chapter outlines the causes and management of hyperglycaemia and hypogly-caemia and Chapter 12 gives advice on the management of diabetes during intercurrent illness.

HYPERGLYCAEMIA

Minor elevations of the blood glucose level outwith the normal range for non-diabetics are almost the rule for diabetic patients, especially if the plasma glucose is measured shortly after eating. Such elevations do not produce any acute problem though they may obviously lead to longer term tissue damage and some of the complications of long-standing diabetes. Only if the blood glucose is consistently elevated above about 15 mmol/l would one become concerned about the short term effects of the hyperglycaemia.

Hyperglycaemia is always due to insulin deficiency, though this deficiency may be absolute, as in the case of the insulin dependent diabetic patient omitting his injected insulin dose, or relative, as in the case of a patient (insulin dependent or non-insulin dependent) failing to respond to the demand for extra insulin posed by steroid therapy, the stress response to intercurrent illness or simple dietary excess. While this distinction may at first appear to be of only academic interest it is vital to appreciate that, while dietary or drug manipulation may be helpful in the latter case, only an increase in the injected dose will resolve the problems in the former case.

Clinical features

The common clinical features of hyperglycaemia are mostly due to the osmotic diuretic effect of glycosuria producing increased urine volume (polyuria) and consequent dehydration and thirst (polydipsia). Urinary symptoms are very prominent in the elderly but may frequently be ignored by patients and doctors who may confuse polyuria and nocturia with urinary frequency and ascribe the symptoms to urinary tract infection or prostatic hypertrophy. This distinction can usually be made clinically, but a simple test for glycosuria can reliably exclude diabetes as a cause of the symptom. Glycosuria may lead to urinary tract infection and so, even in patients with typical symptoms of infection, testing the urine for glucose is important.

Often elderly patients with urinary problems will present not with typical polyuria but with urgency or even incontinence, the bladder sphincter being unable to cope with the large urine volumes being produced. Urinalysis is mandatory in the investigation of any such patient, but it should be remembered that even if a patient is known to have diabetes, sustained absence of glycosuria means that hyperglycaemia and osmotic diuresis are not contributing to the symptomatology and that other investigation is required.

Thirst in elderly patients is often less complained of than in the younger age group. Blame is often laid on diuretic therapy or anti-cholinergic drugs for this symptom and, while these agents may frequently be responsible, hyperglycaemia should also be considered. Simple urinalysis for glucose is the only test that is required, for the thirst always accompanies polyuria due to glycosuria. Excess thirst often leads to the drinking of lemonade, beer or other sugar-containing drinks which may significantly worsen the hyperglycaemia and the consequent symptoms. Exclusion of diabetes is essential before such drinks are advised for the thirsty patient. Some older patients, especially those with restricted independence and those on diuretic therapy, are unable to maintain an adequate fluid intake to keep pace with the osmotic diuresis and may become markedly dehydrated. In an insulin dependent patient this dehydration will usually parallel the development of typical diabetic ketoacidosis but in non-insulin dependent patients the blood glucose may rise to very high levels ($> 100 \, \text{mmol/l}$) without the development of ketosis or acidosis. With severe dehydration and very high blood glucose levels patients become progressively more drowsy and confused and are hence progressively less able to maintain their fluid intake. The diagnosis of this syndrome of hyperosmolar non-ketotic coma (HONK) should be considered in any patient who becomes drowsy or confused, especially if there is dehydration or a history of thirst.

Aetiology

The most common cause of hyperglycaemia in a previously well-controlled diabetic patient is the development of an intercurrent illness such as an infection or a vascular incident (Chapter 12). The physiological response to such a stress leads to markedly increased secretion of hormones which antagonize the actions of insulin and lead to elevation of the plasma glucose.

Major dietary excess, especially the consumption of raw sugar, can lead to severe hyperglycaemia, as can omission or substantial dose reduction of oral hypoglycaemic agents or insulin. The natural history of the disease process in diabetes may lead to a decline in endogenous insulin secretion or increase in insulin resistance, in turn producing a need for either an oral hypoglycaemic agent or insulin therapy.

Investigation

The investigation of the hyperglycaemic patient can largely be done without reference to a specialist laboratory, for the two most important investigations are the blood glucose itself (easily and adequately measured by reagent strips, with or without a reflectance meter) and testing for ketonuria (using reagent tablets or test strips). The absence of ketonuria excludes significant upset in the acid–base balance due to diabetes and further biochemical assessment is not required. Additional investigations may be suggested by the findings of the mandatory full physical examination, which may reveal a cause for the hyperglycaemia such as a chest or urinary tract infection or a cerebro-vascular incident.

Management

If investigation shows the patient to have severe hyperglycaemia (> 25 mmol/l), suggestive of HONK, or significant ketonuria with possible impending ketoacidosis, then prompt referral to hospital for further assessment and management is necessary. Management of ketoacidosis in the elderly is broadly similar to management in younger patients though fluid replacement must be more cautious. Patients presenting with or developing ketoacidosis at any age will usually require insulin treatment thereafter.

Management of HONK involves the cautious correction of the fluid deficit, with parallel insulin treatment of the very marked hyperglycaemia. Mortality in these patients is very high (up to 50%), often due to thrombotic problems accompanying the markedly hyperosmolar state and may possibly be reduced by anticoagulation. Patients developing HONK are usually very insulin sensitive and in the long term can often be managed without insulin, by diet therapy and perhaps oral hypoglycaemic agents in addition.

Assuming that these severe forms of hyperglycaemic metabolic upset have been excluded, the management of hyperglycaemia involves consideration of two main areas, first treatment of the underlying cause, if one can be identified, and secondly management of the elevated blood sugar.

Management of the elevated blood glucose will vary according to the treatment being currently used and is outlined in the list below.

Therapeutic manipulation in the management of hyperglycaemia

Present treatment	*Action if hyperglycaemic*
Diet alone	Check dietary compliance
	THEN

	Add oral hypoglycaemic agent – sulphonylurea if underweight or normal weight and Metformin if obese (and there is no contra-indication)
Diet and sulphonylurea	Check diet and drug compliance THEN Increase sulphonylurea dose by 50–100% (or to maximum recommended dose) THEN Add Metformin (if there is no contraindication) THEN Change to insulin therapy
Diet and Metformin	Check diet and drug compliance. Stop Metformin if patient ill THEN Add sulphonylurea and increase dose as above THEN Change to insulin therapy
Diet and insulin	Check diet and insulin compliance THEN Increase insulin dose by 10–20%. Increase further as dictated by plasma glucose

It is important to realize that for many medical problems such as vascular stroke and myocardial infarction there is evidence to suggest that recovery from the primary problem can be influenced by the level of blood sugar control and that management of diabetes is therefore important in reducing both morbidity and mortality in diabetic patients with other illnesses. If the requirement for increased doses of oral hypoglycaemic agents or insulin is due to an intercurrent illness it usually resolves; it is therefore important that the treatment is modified again after the acute problem has settled if later difficulties with hypoglycaemia are to be avoided.

Sometimes hyperglycaemia may be an indication that the existing form of treatment is no longer adequate and a patient may need to move from diet therapy alone to diet and oral hypoglycaemic agent, or from oral hypoglycaemic agent to insulin therapy. In an elderly patient the decision to start insulin may be made with understandable reluctance, but if the patient has significant symptoms due to hyperglycaemia, or is losing weight, then there is no choice.

Conclusions

A sensible approach to the hyperglycaemic patient allows one to identify readily those patients in whom the metabolic upset is potentially serious and who require intensive therapy and permits a rational approach to the management of patients in whom the metabolic upset is less severe. In all patients the possibility of a significant underlying medical problem must be borne continually in mind.

HYPOGLYCAEMIA

Hypoglycaemia is defined as a plasma glucose of less than 2.5 mmol/l, irrespective of the presence or absence of symptoms. It is usually confined to patients taking drugs which enhance insulin secretion from the pancreas (the sulphonylureas) or taking exogenous insulin. While most professionals involved in the care of diabetic patients accept hypoglycaemia as an inevitable consequence of the treatment, being a simple extension of the therapeutic action of the drugs involved, many patients live in fear of hypoglycaemia. Even mild hypoglycaemia can lead to falls at home and serious fractures, while more severe hypoglycaemia can produce coma, hypothermia and even death in elderly patients living alone.

Clinical features

The clinical features of hypoglycaemia depend both on whether it is acute or chronic and on the response of an individual patient to the stimulus of hypoglycaemia.

Acute hypoglycaemia

This most commonly occurs if food ingestion is reduced, delayed or omitted after taking injected insulin or a sulphonylurea. The timing of the onset of hypoglycaemia depends on the time action of the drug involved; being much shorter with potent sulphonylureas and soluble insulin than with the longer-lasting insulins. The symptoms of hypoglycaemia are controlled by the autonomic nervous system. Initially there is hunger and occasional slight nausea. Later, typical 'fight-or-flight' symptoms of agitation, sweating, pallor and tachycardia develop. As the autonomic symptoms become more marked, symptoms due to insufficient glucose supply to the brain (neuroglycopaenia) begin with irritability, confusion and either agitation or drowsiness developing. If the blood glucose level continues to fall, the neuroglycopaenia becomes more severe and coma will develop, sometimes with associated generalized epileptiform seizures due to severe neuroglycopaenia. Focal neurological signs, such as a hemiparesis or hemiplegia, can also occur in patients with severe neuroglycopaenia, and hypoglycaemia should always be borne in mind as a possible cause of such signs in a diabetic patient.

Elderly patients with autonomic neuropathy may quickly progress to neuroglycopaenia because of the lack of early warning symptoms. A similar situation is seen in patients taking non-selective beta-adrenoceptor blocking drugs, which largely abolish the autonomic symptoms of hypoglycaemia (Chapter 9).

Nocturnal hypoglycaemia may occur unrecognized over a long period and can produce problems such as nocturnal incontinence or confusion. It is rarely seen with sulphonylureas but can occur with longer-acting insulins. The clinical pointers are marked morning headache and, in some patients, morning hyperglycaemia due to increased counter-regulatory hormone secretion overnight.

Chronic hypoglycaemia

This occurs mostly in patients taking long-acting insulins and long-acting sulphonylureas, the blood glucose being at chronically low levels but never falling to levels sufficiently low to produce the acute symptoms and signs outlined above. The clinical presentation is often with mild confusion, like early dementia, or progressive impairment of mobility but no evidence of any focal neurological deficit. The diagnosis can easily be reached by measuring the blood glucose, especially pre-prandially.

Aetiology

Acute hypoglycaemia is almost always due to insulin excess, either absolute in the patient who receives more than their usual dose of injected insulin or oral sulphonylurea (or has an enhanced effect from the usual dose), or relative in the patient who takes their usual dose of hypoglycaemic medication and who consumes less carbohydrate than usual, exercises more vigorously than usual or has reduced levels of counter-regulatory hormones. Only rarely is hypoglycaemia due to other agents (e.g. alcohol) which have a direct hypoglycaemic action.

Overdosage with insulin may be deliberate, in a suicide or para-suicide attempt, or accidental. The latter is surprisingly common as patients of all ages, but especially older patients, may absentmindedly take the wrong dose (or the correct dose at the wrong time). In addition, elderly patients may have difficulty in drawing insulin accurately into a syringe due to co-existing arthritis, neuro-muscular disease or poor vision and can easily administer an accidental overdose. The effects of a usual dose of insulin are rarely increased acutely but failing renal function for whatever cause will impair the metabolism of insulin and can lead to hypoglycaemia while taking a previously well tolerated insulin dose.

Overdosage with sulphonylurea drugs may also be deliberate but is most often accidental due to simple error, forgetfulness or confusion. A change in the unit dose in an individual tablet may also lead to accidental overdosage (e.g. substitution of 5 mg tablets for 2.5 mg tablets). The effects of a dose of a sulphonylurea drug may be enhanced acutely by the simultaneous administration of any drug which displaces the highly protein bound sulphonylureas from their protein binding sites. Drugs implicated include coumarin anticoagulants (warfarin), phenylbutazone and sulphonamide antibiotics. More chronically, the effects of sulphonylurea drugs may be enhanced if there is impairment of metabolism or excretion, this problem being most commonly seen with the long-acting drug chlorpropamide, whose elimination may be very substantially slowed in the presence of renal impairment, leading to drug accumulation and hypoglycaemia.

Probably the most common cause of hypoglycaemia is failure to take adequate carbohydrate following administration of a hypoglycaemic drug. A meal may be delayed due to external circumstances or a patient may forget to take a snack or, sometimes, the important link between the drug and food has not been appreciated so that the patient takes the drug by the clock rather than according to his or her food pattern. Often the problem is compounded by the patient exercising more than usual by, for example, undertaking a shopping trip which leads to increased glucose metabolism due to extra exercise and also leads to lunch being delayed, the combination of circumstances producing hypoglycaemia. Even vigorous housework (e.g. spring cleaning or gardening) can cause the blood glucose to fall to hypoglycaemic levels. Reduced levels of some of the hormones which normally antagonize the action of insulin (growth hormone and cortisol) are seen in patients with untreated hypoadrenalism (Addison's disease) or hypopituitarism. These diseases are rare causes of hypoglycaemia but must be borne in mind if a previously stable patient has inexplicable hypoglycaemic attacks.

Several drugs other than insulin and the sulphonylureas

have been reported to cause hypoglycaemia, the mechanism being unclear but not usually related to increased insulin secretion. Salicylates and tetracycline have been implicated but easily the most frequent other drug causing hypoglycaemia is alcohol. Alcohol produces hypoglycaemia by reducing the hepatic glycogen stores and also by reducing hepatic glucose production and can lead to hypoglycaemia even in the absence of other hypoglycaemic drugs. In combination with either insulin or other sulphonylureas severe hypoglycaemia can occur and may be very difficult to treat.

Chronic hypoglycaemia is usually due to over-zealous administration of the long-acting sulphonylureas, especially in patients in whom elimination of the drug is impaired. Long-acting insulins may also lead to chronic hypoglycaemia but this is much less common.

Management

The treatment of hypoglycaemia involves management of the acute problem, identification of the cause and prevention of recurrence. If the hypoglycaemic patient is able to take fluids or food orally then sugar-containing food or drinks should be given (not unsweetened tea or 'diabetic' foods). Recovery is usually swift (5–15 minutes) but headache may persist for longer. If the patient is unable to take fluids then parenteral therapy with either Glucagon (1 mg intravenous (iv) or intramuscular (im) or subcutaneous (sc)) or dextrose (25 g iv) is necessary. The latter works very rapidly but Glucagon takes 5–20 minutes to have its full effect. If the patient fails to recover in the expected time, the blood glucose should be checked. If it is still low then further parenteral therapy is required but if it is normal or elevated then other causes of impaired consciousness, either related to hypoglycaemia, such as cerebral oedema or a post-ictal state, or unrelated, such as a cerebrovascular incident or drug overdose, must be considered. There is no place for continuing to administer glucose once a normal blood glucose has been achieved for excessive glucose administration can lead to hyperosmolar hypergly-caemic states replacing hypoglycaemia.

Once the patient has recovered from the acute episode, it is essential to make sure that the hypoglycaemia does not recur shortly thereafter, a situation which can easily arise if the patient has taken too much medium or long-acting insulin or long-acting sulphonylurea. If possible, the patient should not be left alone until all risk of recurrent hypoglycaemia has past. Regular carbohydrate ingestion should be encouraged during this period. An effort to establish the cause of the attack should be made by enquiring about drug dose and time of adminis-tration, food ingestion, physical activity and other medication. Often no precise cause can be established, making prevention of recurrence rather difficult.

Appropriate moves to avoid a recurrrence of hypoglycaemia depend on the apparent cause. Simple education and advice about timing of meals, drug dosage and effects of exercise may be adequate; if physical disability makes insulin dosage difficult then aids such as syringe magnifiers, injection guns and 'pen' injection devices may be helpful and still maintain independence. If mental impairment or confusion is a problem then simplification of the treatment regimen (e.g. a single daily dose of drug) or regular supervision of therapy may be necessary.

In view of the potential risks of hypoglycaemia in elderly patients, a pragmatic approach to the level of glycaemic control which one aims to achieve is always required. If significant hypoglycaemia occurs, especially in a patient living alone, then the dose of hypoglycaemic medication will almost always be best reduced, at least temporarily, unless a clear non-recurring cause for the hypoglycaemic episode has been established. Such dose reduction should usually be by about 50% of the daily dose of sulphonylurea drug or 10–20% of the dose of insulin likely to have produced the hypoglycaemia. Diabetic control should be carefully checked in the next few days so that further dosage adjustments, up or down, can be made.

Conclusions

Hypoglycaemia is a real risk to diabetic patients of all ages, but especially elderly patients and should therefore always be taken seriously. Treatment of the acute situation must always be seen as the beginning of the management of the problem and not as an end in itself, as prevention of recurrence is vital.

11
COMPLICATIONS OF DIABETES

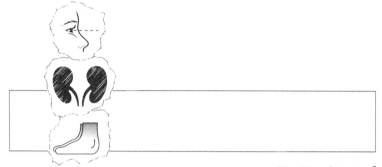

F. I. Caird

The complications of diabetes are important for two reasons: (1) many of them are, up to a point, preventable by strict control of diabetes, and (2) their consequences, such as blindness, kidney failure, and lower limb amputation, are obvious causes of major disability. This is the most important reason, apart from the control of symptoms, for attempting a strict control of diabetes in elderly diabetic patients. In the elderly patient, however, the significance of the complications may be difficult to assess because it is not easy to disentangle them from the other causes of similar states of affairs.

OCULAR COMPLICATIONS

The ocular complications of diabetes are important because as many as 10% of those in whom diabetes is discovered over the age of 70 present with an ocular disorder, most often cataract. The routine testing for diabetes of elderly patients in oph-thalmological clinics is thus a worthwhile procedure. Although diabetic retinopathy is the cause of 7% of newly registered blindness over the age of 65, as many as 10% of blind elderly people have diabetes. The presence of diabetic retinopathy is related in part to the age at onset of the disease, since it appears to be more common in the elderly than in young patients, and very critically to the duration of diabetes. The chances of its developing are of the same order in elderly patients as in younger, and approximately 50% of patients of all ages have retinopathy after 15 years. The relation to control has been established in several studies, and is as easy to demonstrate in elderly patients as in young ones. There is some evidence that the degree of control of the first few years after diagnosis may be especially important, and that this applies to patients whose onset is after, as well as before, the age of 60.

The patterns of retinal involvement in diabetic retinopathy are different from those seen in middle-aged or younger patients. Proliferative retinopathy is the name given to the development of new vessels on the surface of the retina and in front of it, with its high risk of precipitation of blindness from vitreous haemorrhage and retinal detachment from fibrosis.

This form of retinopathy is rare in patients over 70; in them the predominant pathology in the retina is exudative in type, but in so far as the macula is involved (maculopathy), visual impairment or blindness frequently result. The rate of progression of retinopathy, and so the chances of blindness, increase with age; in patients who are over the age of 60 when their diabetes is diagnosed nearly 40% of those who have or who develop retinopathy will suffer from moderate to severe bilateral visual loss within 5 years. In the great majority of these involvement of the macula is the cause.

The principal problem in most of the varieties of maculopathy is leakage from damaged capillaries. This can be difficult to see with the ophthalmoscope, but investigation by fluorescein angiography will establish the exact magnitude and position of the lesions. This involves the intravenous injection of fluorescein-filled capillaries and photographing the leakage from them.

These lesions are treatable by laser photocoagulation, and controlled trials have shown definitely that in many of the varieties of maculopathy it can at least protect vision, and prevent deterioration. The treatment is inconvenient for the patient and time-consuming for both patient and doctor. At this stage, improved control of diabetes does not retard progression of the ocular complications. The principal problem therefore becomes that of screening diabetic patients for retinopathy and offering treatment to those found to have it. Probably the most satisfactory method is the regular examination of the eyes by a competent examiner (say annually), at a specialist clinic. The recently developed non-mydriatic retinal camera, which, as its name implies, dispenses with the need for dilatation of the pupil, is a help in this regard. Any drop in visual acuity at any time which is not obviously due to cataract should lead to referral to an ophthalmologist who is in a position to carry out photocoagulation. The finding of asymptomatic retinopathy should also lead to the same management.

The second major ocular complication of diabetes is cataract. It appears that lens opacities by themselves are no more common in elderly diabetic patients than in non-diabetics, but that operations for cataract are three or four times more common, probably because cataract advances more rapidly in diabetic patients. Both lens opacities and cataract extraction are more common in diabetic women than in men. The appearance and treatment of cataract in elderly diabetic patients are no different to that in non-diabetics, and the indications for operation are the same – moderate diminution of visual acuity in both eyes or severe diminution in one. The operations performed do not differ, and the presence of stable diabetes should never deter or delay the decision to operate if this is indicated. Management of the diabetes before and after operation should be in the hands of a physician experienced in diabetes.

The visual results after operation are the same as in non-diabetics when there is no retinopathy: 80% gain a visual acuity of 6/12 or better, and 5–10% suffer a poor result with a visual acuity of less than 6/60. If there is retinopathy only one-third achieve a good result, and one-third have a poor result, though even in the presence of quite severe retinopathy and even when there is no great improvement of visual acuity, an elderly diabetic patient may still gain a truly worthwhile result from operation.

KIDNEY DISEASES

Exactly as with retinopathy, diabetic renal disease increases with frequency with increasing duration of diabetes, but in old age may also be diagnosed at or soon after the diagnosis of diabetes. The principal clinical manifestation is proteinuria, which is of course in no way specific. Oedema is not unusual, but the blood pressure is rarely greatly raised. At least 80% of those with diabetic renal disease show diabetic retinopathy. The progression of the disease is, on average, slow, and death from co-existing coronary artery disease is more common than that from renal failure. If significant impairment of renal function is present, all drugs, particularly those excreted by the kidney, should be used with caution. In some severe cases, particularly those aged less than 75 years, chronic ambulatory peritoneal dialysis (CAPD) may be worthwhile considering.

NEUROLOGICAL DISORDERS

The classification of the neurological complications of diabetes is difficult, but it is useful to make a simple distinction between a symmetrical, largely sensory, subacute or chronic neuropathy, and a group of asymmetrical, largely motor, often painful, acute conditions. A third group of conditions is created by involvement of the autonomic nervous system.

Symmetrical sensory neuropathy is usually a complication of long-standing diabetes. It may be difficult to diagnose in elderly people because of the high frequency of abnormal neurological signs in elderly subjects without diabetes (e.g. absence of the ankle jerks). Loss of light touch and pain sense in the feet is evidence of a significant neuropathy, and this involvement of the feet in sensory loss plays a very important part in the production of perforating ulceration of the feet (Chapter 8). Pain at night and tenderness in the calves are unusual in elderly people. The management of this type of neuropathy in old age consists largely in protection of the feet from ill-fitting shoes and other forms of trauma. There is no evidence that B-group vitamins are of value.

The variety of motor neuropathy called diabetic amyotrophy requires recognition because its prognosis is very different from that of sensory neuropathy which progresses slowly and does not recover, while amyotrophy characteristically does. The most common clinical presentation is of an elderly patient with a short previous history of diabetes, or even none at all, who develops, over a period of weeks or months, pain, weakness and wasting, first in one thigh and then in the other; there may be gross difficulty in walking. There is no sensory loss unless a sensory neuropathy is present simultaneously; changes in the reflexes reflect muscle wasting. Hyperglycaemia and glycosuria are apparent. The condition usually progresses for some weeks or months, remains static for a further period of a few months, and then slowly improves, usually with complete and permanent recovery of motor power (but not of sensory loss if that is present) in 12–18 months. Most physicians would regard diabetic amyotrophy as an important indication for strict control of diabetes in elderly patients, though it must be admitted that there is relatively little evidence that this greatly affects the outcome in terms of rapidity or completeness of recovery.

When there is involvement of the autonomic nervous system it is often widespread, and tends to occur in those with severe sensory neuropathy. Denervation of the baroreceptor reflexes causes postural hypotension, and the episodes of syncope on standing which result must be distinguished from hypoglycaemic attacks. The diagnosis is made by recording the blood pressure in the standing as well as the lying position, and by the occurrence of symptoms when the blood sugar is not low. Full length elastic stockings and fludrocortisone will assist in controlling this most troublesome symptom.

Disorder of the bowel and bladder is also often seen. Diabetic diarrhoea presents with episodic or continuous diarrhoea, often preceded by loud borborygmi and accompanied by nocturnal incontinence of faeces. Nutrition is well preserved. This distressing condition is thought to be due to bacterial contamination of the small bowel and responds in the majority of cases to antibiotic treatment with tetracycline and metronidazole.

Involvement of the bladder is probably more common than is recognized. It results in a bladder which is dilated and atonic. Factors leading to immobility such as surgical operations and fractures not infrequently precipitate retention of urine. Temporary catheterization and treatment of any urinary infection present often results in functional improvement, but operative treatment by bladder neck resection may be necessary.

VASCULAR DISEASE

The diabetic patient is particularly susceptible to atherosclerosis in any of its forms. Myocardial infarction may present as disordered diabetes, and has a high mortality. The elderly diabetic patient with stroke does not differ in his management from the non-diabetic, but peripheral vascular disease and lesions of the feet are a most important cause of morbidity and of prolonged admission to hospital of elderly diabetic patients. Three elements are involved, either singly or in combination: ischaemia, neuropathy and sepsis. Accurate assessment of the contribution of each is essential for proper management. Ischaemic lesions include both massive gangrene from major arterial occlusion and gangrene of individual toes resulting from pressure or trauma in the presence of local vascular disease. The foot is cold with atrophic and hairless skin, and has a temperature gradient at some point, usually in the calf. The pulses will be impossible to feel, but a swollen but non-ischaemic foot may make for considerable difficulty in deciding whether the pulses are truly absent. There are two common neuropathic lesions: blisters on the toes which rupture to give superficial gangrenous patches and shallow granulating ulcers, and ulceration below the first metatarso-phalangeal joint, which often extends into the joint and sometimes results in the formation of an abscess in the sole of the foot. The ulcer may be covered by a patch of hyperkera-totic skin, and this may mask the seriousness of the underlying state of affairs. The foot is warm and the pulses are usually palpable. Septic lesions may complicate either ischaemia or neuropathy, and X-rays of the feet may show extensive bone destruction.

The principal measures are preventive, and are considered in detail in Chapter 8. Simple foot hygiene, proper footwear, avoidance of damaging extremes of heat and cold, cessation of smoking (which can be insisted upon most strongly in this situation) and regular attendance at the chiropodist are all essential. Neuropathic blisters will heal with rest and anti-biotics, but if there is bone necrosis and abscess formation, surgical treatment and drainage of the abscess is necessary.

Considerable judgement is needed to decide the best course of treatment for ischaemic lesions. Prolonged hospitalization may follow an even minor amputation. The late mortality of patients requiring a high amputation is considerable, though much of this is due to coronary artery disease rather than directly to vascular disease in the leg. However, as many as a quarter of all elderly diabetic patients in whom one amputation is necessary come to a second one before they die.

INFECTIONS

There is an excess prevalence of tuberculosis among diabetic patients of all ages, and it remains reasonable for a chest X-ray to be carried out on all newly discovered diabetic patients, and on all those admitted to hospital. Tuberculosis may precipitate ketosis in elderly patients, and they certainly should not be allowed to leave hospital after an episode of ketosis without a chest X-ray.

Other infections (e.g. of the urine) are probably more common in diabetic patients, but antibiotic therapy and control of the diabetes (which is often disordered by the infection) are highly effective.

12

MANAGEMENT OF INTERCURRENT ILLNESS

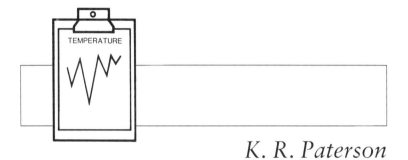

K. R. Paterson

INTERCURRENT ILLNESS

The diabetic patient is no less prone to minor and major non-diabetic medical problems than the non-diabetic patient, but the presence of diabetes may lead to additional management problems. The physiological response to stress, such as an illness, leads to increased circulating levels of growth hormone, cortisol and catecholamines, all hormones which antagonize the actions of insulin and tend to produce hyperglycaemia. In the non-diabetic individual there are also increased circulating levels of insulin which serve to counterbalance the increase in anti-insulin hormones, but this increase in endogenous insulin cannot occur in the truly insulin dependent patient (who has virtually no residual endogenous insulin secretion) and is often inadequate in the non-insulin dependent patient, who may require drug therapy to achieve adequate insulin production even in the absence of intercurrent illness.

In a diabetic patient, even a minor illness such as a viral upper respiratory infection or mild gastroenteritis will tend to lead to hyperglycaemia. Often the patient has a reduced appetite due to the illness and may feel nauseated and unwilling to eat and there is great temptation for all concerned (patient, relative, nurse or doctor) to reduce the dose of insulin or sulphonylurea on the grounds that food ingestion will be less. This is almost always the *wrong* course of action, as the body's need is usually for more insulin in spite of reduced food intake; reducing the dose of hypoglycaemic drug allows the blood sugar, already rising, to rise further and can often lead to metabolic decompensation, either diabetic ketoacidosis or HONK (Chapter 10).

Management of intercurrent illness involves initial assessment by doctor, nurse or patient and then appropriate changes in therapy.

Assessment

Assessment of a diabetic patient with respect to the nature of the intercurrent illness differs little from the non-diabetic. The diabetic state should be assessed by measurement of blood glucose (or urine glucose if blood glucose testing is not possible) and testing for ketonuria. A finding of a very high blood glucose (> 25 mmol/l) or more than minimal ketonuria is an indication for prompt hospitalization as major metabolic decompensation may be imminent. In addition, severe vomiting such as to prevent the taking of any food or fluid and unrelieved by usual antiemetic therapy, will usually also force hospital admission.

If there is only minor ketonuria (such as one normally sees in any unwell patient) and the blood sugar is not too high then treatment at home is possible.

Management

Treatment of the intercurrent illness is little affected by the presence of diabetes (except for some limitations on drugs used, Chapter 9) and should proceed along conventional lines. If the patient is unable to take solid food due to vomiting or difficulty swallowing then adequate carbohydrate may be given in the form of liquids (e.g. milk, fizzy drinks etc) or semi-solids (egg soups, icecream). Every effort should be made to maintain the usual carbohydrate intake in all patients, though this is most important in insulin dependent patients who are at greatest risk of metabolic decompensation if carbohydrate intake is reduced. Patients taking diet therapy alone often cope with mild intercurrent illness without too many problems but some may need a sulphonylurea drug in the short term. Patients on oral hypoglycaemic agents or insulin should have their usual dose continued or even increased if the plasma glucose is elevated (see list, p. 73–74).

The biguanide drug Metformin should not be given during intercurrent illness, especially if there is hypotension or reduced peripheral perfusion (e.g. after an acute myocardial infarction), as there is a significant risk of lactic acidosis. (Chapter 5). Metformin should be withdrawn and a sulphonylurea agent used temporarily.

The crucial importance of frequent monitoring of diabetes

(by either blood or urine tests) must be emphasized to the patient and to others involved in his or her management. An acute illness is a dynamic situation and therapy may need to be changed on a day to day basis to cope with the changing metabolic state. Often the ill patient is not sufficiently motivated to keep a close watch on their diabetes or may be unable to monitor it adequately because of the effects of the acute illness, so whenever possible a third party, either a relative or health professional, should also keep a close check on the diabetes.

Once the patient has recovered from the acute illness it is important that diabetic therapy is reassessed, as the dose of drug will normally require to be reduced over 1–2 weeks as the levels of anti-insulin hormones fall. Failure to adequately monitor diabetes in the convalescence after an acute illness can later lead to hypoglycaemia if an increased dose of hypo-glycaemic drug is continued when the need for it has gone.

CONCLUSIONS

Illness in a diabetic patient must be treated vigorously, with frequent review of blood glucose control and changes in diabetic management from day to day. Hyperglycaemia is more of a problem than hypoglycaemia in this setting and, at very least, patients should be told to continue their usual hypoglycaemic therapy. The majority of cases of severe metabolic decompensation in elderly patients are in part attributable to reduction or withdrawal of therapy, an easily avoidable problem.

13

THE ROLE OF THE SPECIALIST NURSE

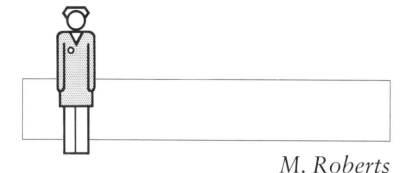

M. Roberts

THE SPECIAL NEEDS OF ELDERLY PATIENTS

The educational needs of the elderly person with diabetes may not be significantly different from those of the younger person. However, the nurse should be aware of the potential problems and complications associated with advancing age which may affect the individual's ability to cope with their disease. In this chapter I will identify the possible difficulties that elderly patients may encounter with education, diet, medication, injections, home monitoring and foot care and discuss the role of the specialist nurse in assessment.

ASSESSMENT

Careful assessment of the diabetic elderly patient is required. Nurses and doctors, particularly those working in hospitals, often have a rather jaundiced view of old age, mainly because their experience of elderly patients gives the impression that this stage of life inevitably results in growing dependence, frailty and mental deterioration. The saying 'you can't teach an old dog new tricks' is the view so often reflected by society. Expectations of health in old age can be low. Such views cause barriers to education and health promotion which the nurse will have to overcome. It is encouraging to find that the majority of elderly people are leading full, independent and active lives and assessment should not be made merely on a patient's chronological age.

The aim of diabetic care is the initiation, establishment and maintenance of diabetic control, the prevention, early detection and treatment of diabetic complications and the retention of a normal lifestyle within the constraints of the disease. The elderly person will require the help, guidance, education and support of the nurse in adapting to the new demands and changes in his life but there is certainly no reason why he should not be an active partner in the making of the decisions affecting his health and wellbeing. The enthusiastic attendance at diabetic education classes show that elderly patients, like any other age group, wish to have an understanding of the disease process affecting them and want to know what contribution they can make to enhance and retain their health. Lack of motivation, by otherwise fit, elderly patients, requires investigation. Some elderly people feel that they are being a 'burden'. Others may take the diagnosis of diabetes too lightly since the non-insulin dependent diabetic is often told he has mild diabetes. Anxiety, denial, fear and underlying social problems will affect the patient's willingness and ability to learn and accept information.

Not all elderly patients will be capable of self management. The specialist nurse will come into contact with patients suffering from other chronic illnesses, affecting mobility and the ability to carry out daily activities. All patients should be encouraged and helped to reach their full potential. The specialist nurse has an important role to play in the support and education of the carers. Less emphasis will be placed on euglycaemia. Relief of symptoms and, in particular, prevention of hypoglycaemia will be the priority. Liaison with other members of the paramedical staff to ensure continuity of care and advice is essential. The longstanding diabetic may have changing needs and requirements as he approaches retirement and the alteration in lifestyle that it imposes. Advancing years, growing frailty and mental decline will all affect the continuing independence of the patient. The specialist nurse is a permanent figure in the life of the diabetic. A genuine interest, accessibility and willingness to listen make the nurse easily approachable, particularly for the diabetic patient who is experiencing difficulty with some aspect of his management. Diabetes is a life-long disorder and the assessment of the patient's needs and educational requirements is an essential and continuing process.

TEACHING ELDERLY DIABETIC PATIENTS

In my own experience I have found elderly patients as capable of learning new skills as anyone else, but obviously it is important to adapt one's teaching method to the needs of the individual. Usually a slower pace is necessary, with attainable short term goals. Information often has to be explained and repeated over several sessions with regular updates. Frequently elderly patients lack confidence in their abilities. Achievement is always rewarded by praise. Patience, encouragement and optimism will inspire the patient to overcome those aspects of his management with which he is having most difficulty. I always try to ensure a calm, unhurried atmosphere in which the patient can feel relaxed and is reassured that he is not taking up the time of the 'busy' nurse. Accuracy is of far greater importance than speed, and those people involved in the care of elderly people, whether they are a nurse, relative or doctor, must resist the temptation to interfere when an elderly person is struggling to master a procedure. Thoughtless intervention, which unfortunately does happen, undermines the patient's confidence and deprives him of success.

Within our Diabetic Department we have various videos and slides to aid our education programmes. Elderly patients, however, tend to prefer to have information communicated to them verbally by the teacher. This, in itself, can pose a special problem since many elderly people are unwilling to admit that they have impaired hearing. For our new type II diabetics we run a series of educational classes which are not only informative for the patient but also give them an opportunity to meet people and to swap views and experiences. Not all patients are suitable for such classes and it may be better for the person who has a hearing difficulty to be seen separately with his family. I always ensure that any education booklets I use are in large, bold print. In general, I always work through pamphlets and booklets with the patient since they often find this helpful and it can prompt some productive discussion. Certainly booklets handed out with little explanation of their content are of little value. One should always take into consideration the fact that some patients may be unable to read. Obviously, it is necessary to discreetly and tactfully establish this fact. I usually ask them to read back some instructions that I have written out for them.

Language difficulties amongst immigrants living in Britain is a frequently encountered problem. Translators should be available, and other members of the patient's family, with a good command of English, will usually prove very helpful and supportive.

The relatives of the elderly person should always be encouraged to attend education sessions. This will help relieve their own anxieties and will give them the necessary information to encourage and assist the diabetic person within the family.

It is important not to overload elderly patients with information since it may leave them feeling helpless and confused. For the newly diagnosed insulin dependent diabetic, or secondary failure, a 'survival package' is all that is necessary in the early days. This package consists of insulin administration (if appropriate), dietary advice, signs, symptoms, cause and action to be taken in the event of hypoglycaemia. For those patients admitted to hospital for stabilization it is important that the specialist nurse maintains a good rapport with the ward team, remembering that they are there at the invitation of the ward sister.

For patients taking insulin for the first time it can often be unrealistic to expect them to cope with their own injections. It can be many months before an elderly person feels confident to carry out injections unsupervized. The district nurses are invaluable for their contribution to the ongoing care and continuation of education. It is extremely important that the specialist nurse liaises and works effectively with nursing colleagues, reviewing the patient and giving help, support and advice when requested.

DIETARY PROBLEMS

It is essential that the diabetic nurse specialist has a sound knowledge of the dietary requirements of the diabetic patient, working in co-operation with the dietician. Close contact with and knowledge of the patient places the nurse in a position to identify problems which threaten the success of any dietary advice.

Elderly people are particularly vulnerable to feelings of

loneliness and depression, perhaps as a consequence of the death of a spouse. Irregular eating habits and even anorexia may develop as a result. Under these circumstances the patient who is taking insulin or oral hypoglycaemics is at risk of becoming hypoglycaemic. For a patient living alone this can be disastrous.

Preparing and eating food is a social event and a patient living alone may be disinclined to prepare food for himself. Poor mobility and reduced dexterity can cause problems in the actual production of a meal. There is an obvious role for the nurse specialist in identifying such problems and mobilizing the necessary resources to prevent a crisis occurring, e.g. Meals on Wheels, lunch clubs, etc.

The occupational therapist will perhaps be of some service to the individual having difficulties in handling awkward kitchen utensils, etc. Misconceptions may arise from the meaning of a 'sugar free' diet and the diabetic may become very limited in the food they select. An elderly woman at our clinic had taken the meaning of 'sugar free' so literally that she had, for some months, been living on cold meat since everything else seemed to contain sugar in some shape or form. It may be worthwhile, at the patient's invitation, to go through their food cupboard identifying those foods that are suitable and pointing out the possible additions that could be made.

Decaying teeth and poor fitting dentures which cause discomfort when chewing can prevent patients eating adequately. It is important that such problems are identified since they can be easily remedied.

Financial difficulties can affect the individual's ability to follow a suitable diet. This may become apparent at a home visit. Liaison with the social worker is often helpful since elderly people are often unaware of the social security benefits available to them.

DIFFICULTIES ENCOUNTERED WITH TABLET AND INSULIN THERAPY

Elderly people often find themselves in the position of swallowing a confusing array of tablets with little idea of when or why they are taking them. Admissions to hospital may result in them being discharged with yet another addition to their medicine cabinet. Busy general wards may have little time to spare in explaining the name, dose and timing of medication to patients. The patient will not have been given the opportunity to take responsibility for their administration. Once home, patients may be unable to read the instructions on the bottle, may have difficulty in, opening childproof containers due to arthritic hands and may be under the misconception that they are on a course of tablets and do not attend their doctors for a repeat prescription. Difficulty with swallowing discourages the patient from continuing with therapy. Failing memory may result in overdosage or underdosage of medication, including insulin. It is important that the nurse ensures that the patient can safely administer the prescribed medication. Confusion often arises when the patient has a number of incomplete containers of the same tablets. One incidence that can be recalled was a man who was asked to bring his medicine bottles along to the clinic since there was some doubt as to whether or not he was complying with this therapy. He brought three containers, one stating Glucophage 500 mg and the other two stating Metformin 500 mg but obviously produced at different pharmaceutical companies. The outcome of this was the patient thought each container held a different type of tablet and felt totally incapable of complying with the instructions on each container which were 'take one tablet three times a day with meals'!

Other members of the household will usually supervise medication administration for those patients having difficulty. For the patient living alone; if after assessment it is thought that it would be dangerous for them to be left unsupervised, it may be necessary to enlist the help of the community nursing officer.

Failing eyesight may cause increasing difficulty for the patient with insulin dependent diabetes. Patients who have been managing admirably well over the years are often unwilling to admit to difficulties. Hypoglycaemia, hyperglycaemia or erratic control may be a consequence of inaccurate insulin dosage. It is well worth reassessing the patient's insulin injection technique throughout his diabetic career. For these patients and for newly diagnosed insulin dependent diabetic patients it is worth investigating the equipment now available for those with visual difficulties in order to maintain their independence. New ideas are developing all the time.

HOME MONITORING – URINE AND BLOOD TESTING

This aspect of care is discussed in Chapter 7. Nurses should be aware of the difficulties that may be encountered in this area, e.g. deteriorating vision, colour blindness or practical difficulties with the technique due to arthritic or unsteady hands.

FOOT CARE

This has been discussed in greater detail in Chapter 8. Diabetic specialist nurses have a significant role to play in teaching the diabetic patient and his family about the importance of foot care. Evidence suggests that improved patient awareness about the need for foot care can greatly reduce the number of amputations occurring.

CONCLUSION

The specialist nurse is an essential member of the diabetic team, maintaining the health, happiness and independence of the elderly diabetic patient. As yet, however, there are few diabetic specialist nurses and, while this situation continues to exist, they must extend their role to encompass the continuing education of other medical and nursing staff in the needs of the elderly diabetic patient.

14
SHARED CARE

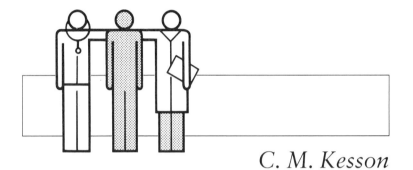

C. M. Kesson

SHARED CARE

Diabetes mellitus is a common chronic disease requiring life-long treatment but, with effective management, the patient can enjoy a full and active lifestyle. A major problem, however, is how to effect satisfactory medical supervision for the large number of patients who suffer from diabetes. It has been estimated that more than 1 in 10 of people aged over 65 may have diabetes, and the elderly population is increasing. In the past 60 years, following the discovery of insulin, a network of hospital based diabetic clinics has evolved and, until recently, many patients who had diabetes were obliged to attend hospital based clinics for supervision of the disease. This was largely because of the perceived difficulty in managing patients receiving insulin therapy. However, the vast majority of elderly diabetics are non-insulin dependent.

It is mainly the increase in non-insulin dependent elderly diabetics which has increased the workload of the clinics over the years, and thus they have become too busy. As a result some of these patients are discharged from the clinic and some surveys show that thereafter they often receive no follow up at all. The clinics are also unpopular with patients for a number of reasons. The inconvenience for the patient travelling sometimes long distances to attend the hospital clinic and the fact that regular visits throughout their lives are required is certainly not a point in, their favour. In addition, at many hospital clinics patients consult different doctors at each visit and when a long-standing diabetic patient consults a very junior doctor, the patient may feel that the visit was not entirely beneficial. In recent years a system of shared care, whereby patients can be supervised intermittently at hospital, but more frequently by their own general practitioners between hospital visits, has emerged.

BENEFITS OF SHARED CARE

There are great benefits, particularly for older patients, who, when visiting their family doctor, are seen by the same doctor and the same nurse each time. They do not have long to wait at each appointment. The cost of travelling is reduced and visits to a familiar general practitioner are less likely to produce anxiety. The system provides greater job satisfaction for the general practitioner who can help to reduce morbidity and endeavour to improve the quality of the patient's life. General practitioners who become involved in shared care of diabetic patients acquire greater skill in their management. From the point of view of hospital staff, the shared care system of diabetic patient management is attractive because the number of patients attending any diabetic clinic is reduced and the hospital physician is free to have a more relaxed and lengthy consultation with the patient at their intermittent visit.

DRAWBACKS OF THE SYSTEM

Communication problems

A shared care system utilizing hospital and general practitioner facilities provides two sites of reference for the diabetic patient. It is essential that good communication between the hospital and the general practitioner is maintained for it is tragic when a diabetic patient has been lost to follow-up and found only years later when irremediable complications are present. Computerization of diabetic patient lists are useful in prevention of such problems but a well thought out, active, two-way communication system between hospital doctor and the primary care doctor must be set up.

Facilities

Hospital diabetic clinics have on-site specialist dietetic and chiropody services and may have special equipment used for early detection of chronic complications. These facilities may be lacking in some general practitioner surgeries and it is crucial that introduction of a shared-care system does not lead to deterioration in the service provided for the patient. A résumé of the facilities required to set up a general practice diabetic mini-clinic is given in the list below.

Necessities for commencing a shared care clinic in general practice

1. An interested general practitioner who is willing to learn;
2. Space and time for the clinic with a regular session set aside. Trying to see patients during ordinary surgery time is not usually satisfactory;
3. Access to the services of a practice nurse or health visitor;
4. A system of record keeping and some method of chasing defaulters;
5. Good liaison with the specialist hospital services;
6. Access to an onsite glucometer and/or local biochemistry facilities and glycosylated haemoglobin measurements.

Loss of expertise

Inevitably if one partner cultivates an expertise in a particular condition then this will lead to them looking after all the diabetic patients in the practice. This is a matter which must be resolved before commencing a clinic. In addition it would require a practice of over 5000 patients to make the clinic a worthwhile exercise, because of the incidence of diabetes in the general population.

CONCLUSION

The institution of a shared care programme for management of diabetic patients can be very worthwhile with benefits obvious to patients, family doctors and hospital doctors alike. One of the main problems with initial efforts in this direction was that patients tended to drop out and were not adequately followed up. However, with the advent of more computer systems, satisfactory recall can be organized from a hospital base. The patients can then be monitored much more frequently than would be possible if all the attendances had to be at a hospital clinic, but the benefit of the facilities available in modern diabetic clinics are not lost to the patients. The system is particularly of value to elderly patients who predominate in any diabetic population.

APPENDIX A
Dietary guidelines for elderly diabetic patients

FOOD ALLOWED

The following foods contain little or no sugar, but protein foods such as meat, fish, eggs and poultry contain both fat and energy and therefore should be eaten in moderation.

Meat	Lean meat, mince, stew, beef, lamb, pork, ham, liver, kidney, cooked or tinned meats. Choose leaner varieties where possible.
Poultry	Chicken, turkey, duck.
Fish	Fresh or frozen, tinned, smoked.
Fats	Butter, margarine, ghee, lard, dripping, oil. Use these sparingly.
Eggs	Fry only occasionally.
Cheese	Use those containing less fat e.g. cottage cheese, edam, gouda, low fat Cheddar and Cheshire, crowdie, camembert.
Fruit	Several portions of any seasonal fresh fruit daily, including apples, bananas, fresh guava, grapefruit, pear, peach, pineapple, oranges, fresh lychees.
Vegetables	Fresh, frozen, raw or pickled (without sugar) Asparagus, artichoke, aubergine, beansprouts,

broccoli, brussel sprouts, cabbage, carrots, cauliflower, celery, chinese leaves, chillies, courgette (zucchini, squash) cucumber, fennel, green beans, leeks, lettuce, marrow, mushrooms, mustard, cress, onions, okra, peas (not processed), peppers, radish, root ginger, spinach, spring onions, swede, tomato, turnip, watercress, vine leaves.

Soups Thin vegetable soup, consommé.

Beverages Tea, coffee, water, soda-water, sugar-free squashes, low-calorie drinks, lemon juice, Bovril, Oxo, Marmite and stock cubes.

Seasonings Salt, pepper, herbs, spices, curry powder, garlic, mustard, tumeric, chilli powder, ground ginger, coriander, oregano, paprika, saffron, tamarind. Food essences and colourings. Gelatine

Sweeteners Saccharine and aspartame sweeteners.

FOODS TO BE AVOIDED

The following foods contain rapidly absorbed sugars and therefore should be avoided.

Sugar,
dextrose,
glucose,
glucose drinks,
glucose sweets,
sherberts,
jam,
marmalade,
honey,
treacle,
syrup,
lemon curd,
mincemeat,

marzipan,
Turkish delight,
sweets,
chocolate,
peppermints,
chewing gum,
chocolate biscuits,
sweet biscuits,
buns,
cakes,
pies and pastries,
shortbread,
lemonade,

fruit squashes,
fizzy drinks,
milk shake syrups
  or powder,
bottled sauces,
sweet chutneys,
tinned fruit in
  syrup,
sweetened
  condensed milk,
sugar coated
  breakfast
  cereals.

FOODS WHICH CONTAIN CARBOHYDRATE

Foods in italics are high in fibre or low in fat and are therefore recommended. Carbohydrate-containing foods should be taken regularly at each meal.

Bread	Bread, rolls, baps, croissants, pitta bread, bagel, *wholemeal bread and rolls, wholemeal pitta bread*, chapatis.
Biscuits	Plain biscuits, e.g. *digestive biscuits bran biscuits, wholemeal crackers and crispbreads, oatcakes*, rich tea biscuits, cream crackers, crispbreads and water biscuits, plain matzo crackers, plain scones, currant buns (not sugar coated).
Cereals	Cornflour, custard, sago, tapioca, barley, white semolina, rice, *wholemeal semolina*, flour, *wholemeal flour*, Rice crispies, cornflakes, Special K, *all bran, Shredded Wheat, Weetabix, puffed wheat, branflakes, unsweetened muesli, porridge*.
Pasta	Spaghetti, macaroni, noodles, *choose wholemeal varieties*.
Legumes	*Peas, beans, lentils (dhal)*.
Vegetables	*Sweetcorn*, yam, Chinese mushrooms, plantain, potatoes (boiled, *baked in jacket*, mashed, chipped, potato crisps).
Milk and yoghurt	Fresh, *skimmed or semi-skimmed low-fat yoghurt*, fruit flavoured yoghurt, *unsweetened fruit yoghurt*.
Fruit	Canned in its own juice (see foods allowed) natural fruit juice, jelly, ice-cream
Soups	*Lentil, pea soup, vegetable or Scotch broth*.
Miscellaneous	Black pudding, sausage, haggis, fish fingers, samosas, sausage rolls, pies, pastry, pakora (bhaji), pickled vegetables in vinegar (no sugar added).

FOOD EXCHANGES LIST FOR ELDERLY DIABETIC PATIENTS

The following list of foods contain 10 g carbohydrate i.e. 1 exchange. It represents only a small part of the exchange lists available for diabetics.

Food	*Handy Measure*
Wholemeal bread or white bread	½ large slice or 1 small
Digestive biscuits	1 large
Branflakes/cornflakes	3 heaped tablespoons
Muesli unsweetened	2 level tablespoons
Chapati	1 very thin saucer size
Brown or white rice	2 level tablespoons
Plantain – green, raw	1 small slice
Potato	
boiled	1 small
jacket	1 medium
roast	½ medium
Sweet potato – raw, peeled	1 small slice
Apple – *with skin*	1 small
Apricots – fresh	4 medium
Banana	1 small
Guavas – fresh	1
Mango – fresh	⅓ large
Orange – fresh	1 medium
Pawpaw – fresh	⅙ large
Milk	
fresh, whole	1 glass (200 ml)
semi-skimmed	1 glass (200 ml)
Yoghurt – plain and diet	1 small carton
Sausages – grilled	2 average sized
Scones	1 small

APPENDIX B
Ten basic instructions for patients

1. Take regular exercise, it helps diabetic control;
2. If possible adopt a regular eating pattern;
3. If you become more thirsty have your blood glucose checked;
4. If vomiting occurs seek medical advice without delay;
5. Act quickly when you notice the initial symptoms of hypoglycaemia;
6. Report frequent hypoglycaemia. Diabetes can be controlled without this;
7. If you take insulin, always carry glucose tablets or sweets and an ID card;
8. Never stop insulin;
9. Look after your feet carefully, if you can't manage, get someone to do it for you;
10. Never be frightened or embarrassed to ask for help: better safe than sorry.

APPENDIX C
Useful addresses

British Geriatrics Society,
1 St Andrew's Place,
Regents Park,
London, NW1 4LB, UK

American Geriatrics Society,
770 Lexington Avenue,
Suite 400,
New York, NY 10021, USA

Australian Association of Gerontology,
The Science Centre,
35–43 Clarence St,
Sydney 2000, Australia

New Zealand Geriatric Society,
48 Hood Street,
Dunedin, New Zealand

British Diabetic Association,
10 Queen Anne St,
London, W1M 0BD, UK

American Diabetic Association,
1660 Duke St,
Alexandria, VA 22314, USA

Chest Heart and Stroke Association,
Tavistock House North,
Tavistock Square,
London, WC1W 9JE, UK

Scottish National Federation For the Welfare of the Blind,
8 St Leonard's Bank,
Perth, PH2 8EB, UK

Talking Newspaper Association of the United Kingdom,
68a High St,
Heathfield,
East Sussex, TN21 8JB, UK

Centre for Policy on Ageing,
Nuffield Lodge Stucho,
Regents Park,
London, NW1 4RS, UK

British Association for Services to the Elderly,
3 Keele Farmhouse,
Keele,
Newcastle-under-Lyme, ST5 1AX, UK

British Society for Research on Ageing,
Geigy Unit for Research in Ageing,
Department of Geriatric Medicine,
University Hospital of South Manchester,
Manchester, M20 8LR, UK

Age Concern Scotland,
33 Castle Street,
Edinburgh, EH2 3DN UK

Age Concern England,
60 Pitcairn Road,
Mitcham,
Surrey, CR4 3LL, UK

Diabetes Australia,
QBE Building 33–35 Ainslie Avenue,
Canberra ACT,
PO Box 944, Civic Square ACT 2608,
Australia

Irish Diabetic Association,
82–83 Lower Gardiner Street,
Dublin 1,
Eire

Canadian Diabetes Association,
78 Bond Street,
Toronto,
Ontario M5B 2J8
Canada

New Zealand Diabetes Association,
4 Coquet Street,
PO Box 54,
Oamaru,
New Zealand

Medic Alert Foundation,
11/13 Clifton Terrace,
London N4 3JP, UK

Pharmaceutical companies who provide useful practical educational literature

Servier Laboratories Ltd,
Fulmer Hall,
Windmill Road,
Fulmer,
Slough, SL3 6HH, UK

Sterling–Winthrop Research Laboratories,
Onslow Street,
Guildford,
Surrey, GU1 4YS, UK

Eli Lilly and Company Ltd,
City Wall House,
Basing View,
Basingstoke,
Hampshire, RG21 2LA, UK

Becton Dickinson UK Ltd,
Diabetes Health Care Division,
Between Towns Road,
Cowley,
Oxford, OX4 3LY, UK

Nordisk-UK,
Nordisk House,
Garland Court, Garland Road,
East Grinstead, RH19 1DN, UK

BCL, Boehringer Corporation (London) Ltd,
Boehringer Mannheim House,
Bell Lane, Lewes,
East Sussex, BN7 1LG, UK

Ames Division, Miles Ltd,
PO Box 37,
Stoke Court, Stoke Poges,
Slough, SL2 4LY, UK

Novo Laboratories Ltd,
Ringway House, Bell Road,
Doneshill East, Basingstoke,
Hampshire, RG24 0QB, UK

Suppliers of equipment (injection devices, monitoring equipment etc)

Hypoguard (UK) Ltd,
Dock Lane, Woodbridge,
Suffolk, IP12 1PE, UK

Owen Mumford Ltd,
Brookhill, Woodstock,
Oxon OX7 1TU, UK

Contacta,
TVM (Manchester) Ltd,
9 Bloom Street,
Salford, Lancashire, UK

APPENDIX D
Further reading

This appendix gives the reader some source material from which to gain some more detailed knowledge. When a chapter does not have detailed further reading then information can be gleaned from the more general texts listed under the heading of general background reading.

GENERAL BACKGROUND READING

Krall, L. P. (ed.) (1988) *World Book of Diabetes in Practice* (Vol. 3) Elsevier, Amsterdam.

Ireland, J. T., Thomson, W. S. T. and Williamson, J. (1980) *Diabetes Today*, HM & M Publishers, Aylesbury.

Shaw, M. W. (ed.) (1984), *The Challenge of Ageing*, Churchill Livingstone, Edinburgh.

Brocklehurst, J. C. (ed.) (1985) *Textbook of Geriatric Medicine and Gerontology*, 3rd ed, Churchill Livingstone, Edinburgh.

Ellenburg, M. and Rifkin, H. (eds) (1983) *Diabetes Mellitus*, 3rd ed, Medical Examination Publishing, New York.

Practical Diabetes, Journal for The Diabetes Care Team, The Newbourne Group; Home and Law Publishing Ltd, Hampstead Rd, London NW1 7QQ.

Pathy, M. S. J. (ed.) (1985) *The Principles and Practice of Geriatric Medicine*, John Wiley, Chichester.

Diabetes Care, The Journal of Clinical and Applied Research and Education, American Diabetes Association, Alexandria Va., USA.

Bloom, A. and Ireland, J. (eds) (1980) *A Colour Atlas of Diabetes*, Wolfe Medical Publications Ltd, London.

Care of the Elderly, The Newbourne Group; Home and Law Publishing Ltd, Hampstead Road, London NW1 7QQ.

CHAPTERS 1 AND 2

Mann, J. L., Pyorala, K. and Teuscher, A. (1983) *Diabetes in Epidemiological Perspective*, Churchill Livingstone, Edinburgh.

Levin, M. E. (1982) Diabetes: the geriatric difference, *Geriatrics*, 37(12) 41–45.

Hindson, D. A. (1984) Diagnosis and treatment of diabetes mellitus in *Drug Treatment in the Elderly* (ed. R. E. Vestal) Adis Health Science Press, Sydney.

CHAPTER 3

Knight, P. V. and Kesson, C. M. (1986) Educating the elderly diabetic, *Diabetic Medicine* 3(2) 170–173.

Assal, J. P. and Pernet, A. (1982) Education as part of therapy in (eds) L. P. Krall and K. G. M. M. Abertii, *World Book of Diabetes in Practice*, Excerpta Medica, Amsterdam.

Baksi, A. K., Hide, D. and Giles, G. (eds) (1984) *Diabetes Education*, John Wiley, Chichester.

Assal, J. P., Alivisatos, J. G. and Halimi, D. (eds) (1988) *The

Teaching Letter, Diabetes Education Study Group of The European Association for the Study of Diabetes, Artem, 27 Rue du Pont 92200 Neuilly-Sur-Seine, France.

CHAPTER 4

Thomas, B. (ed.) (1988) *Manual of Dietetic Practice*, British Dietetic Association, Blackwell Scientific, Oxford.

Krause, M. V. and Mahon, L. K. (1984) *Food, Nutrition and Diet Therapy*, 7th ed, Saunders, Philadelphia.

Tarr, S. P., Wenlock, R. W. and Buss, D. H. (1985) *Immigrant Foods*, Second Supplement to McCance and Widdowson's Composition of Food, HMSO, London.

CHAPTER 5

Knight, P. V. (1987) The choice of oral hypoglycaemic agent for the elderly in *Advanced Geriatric Medicine 6*, (eds F. I. Caird and J. G. Evans) P. S. G. Wright, Bristol pp. 151–154.

Knight, P. V., Semple, C. G. and Kesson, C. M. (1986) The use of Metformin in the elderly patient *Journal of Clinical and Experimental Gerontology*, 8(1,2) 51–58.

CHAPTER 7

Martin, B. J., Knight, P. V., Kesson, C. M., O'Donnell, J. R. and Young, R. E. (1984) Glycosylated haemoglobin: its value in screening for diabetes mellitus in the elderly. *Journal of Clinical and Experimental Gerontology*, 6(2) 87–94.

CHAPTER 8

Connor, H. M., Boulton, A. J. M. and Ward, J. D. (eds) (1986) *The Foot in Diabetes*, John Wiley, Chichester.

Faris, I. (1983) *Management of the Diabetic Foot*, Churchill Livingstone, Edinburgh.

CHAPTER 9

Scott, P. J. W. and Caird, F. I. (1986) *Drug-Induced Diseases in the Elderly*, Elsevier, Amsterdam, pp. 37–44 and 155–156.

Chen, M. S., Hindson, D. A. and Vestal, R. E. (1987) Hypoglycaemic agents and the treatment of Diabetes Mellitus in the elderly, in *Clinical Pharmacology in the Elderly*, (ed. C. Swift) Dekker, New York, pp. 581–628.

CHAPTER 11

Caird, F. I. (1980) Management of Diabetes and Its Complications in *Metabolic and Nutritional Disorders in the Elderly*, (eds A. N. Exton-Smith and F. I. Caird) Wright, Bristol, pp. 161–179.

Kennedy, H. and Caird, F. I. (1986) Diabetic retinopathy in *The Eye and its Disorders in the Elderly*, (eds J. Williamson and F. I. Caird) Wright, Bristol, pp. 101–110.

CHAPTER 13

Kinson, J. and Natrass, M. (1984) *Caring for The Diabetic Patient*, Churchill Livingstone, Edinburgh.

INDEX